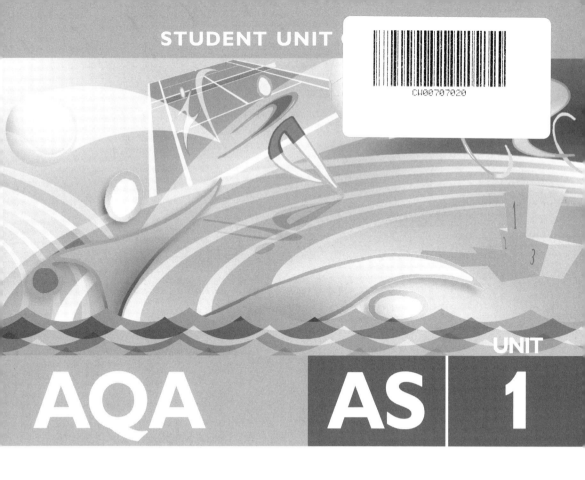

AQA AS UNIT 1

Physical Education

Opportunities for, and the Effects of, Leading a Healthy and Active Lifestyle

Symond Burrows, Michaela Byrne and Sue Young

Philip Allan Updates, an imprint of Hodder Education, an Hachette UK company, Market Place, Deddington, Oxfordshire OX15 0SE

Orders

Bookpoint Ltd, 130 Milton Park, Abingdon, Oxfordshire OX14 4SB
tel: 01235 827720
fax: 01235 400454
e-mail: uk.orders@bookpoint.co.uk
Lines are open 9.00 a.m.–5.00 p.m., Monday to Saturday, with a 24-hour message answering service. You can also order through the Philip Allan Updates website: www.philipallan.co.uk

© Philip Allan Updates 2008

ISBN 978-0-340-94787-6

This Guide has been written specifically to support students preparing for the AQA AS Physical Education Unit 1 examination. The content has been neither approved nor endorsed by AQA and remains the sole responsibility of the authors.

Printed by MPG Books, Bodmin

Hachette UK's policy is to use papers that are natural, renewable and recyclable products and made from wood grown in sustainable forests. The logging and manufacturing processes are expected to conform to the environmental regulations of the country of origin.

Contents

Introduction

■ ■ ■

Content Guidance

Applied exercise physiology

Skill acquisition

Opportunities for participation

■ ■ ■

Questions and Answers

Introduction

About this guide

This unit guide is written to help you prepare for the AQA PE Unit 1 test. **Section A** of the Unit 1 test examines the AS theoretical content of three aspects of PE, namely:

- applied exercise physiology
- skill acquisition
- opportunities for participation

The question in **Section B** relates to the practical aspects of applied skill and fitness and training, which are outlined in Unit 2 of the AS specification.

This **Introduction** provides advice on how to use the unit guide and some suggestions for effective revision. Each aspect of the specification required for the Unit 1 test is covered in the **Content Guidance**. The **Questions and Answers** section provides examples of questions from various topic areas, together with student answers and examiner's comments on how these could have been improved.

The specification

Unit 1 is about the opportunities for, and the effects of, leading a healthy and active lifestyle. The specification describes the aspects of PE that you need to learn. If you do not have a copy of the specification, ask your teacher for one or download it from the AQA website, **www.aqa.org.uk**. The examiners will pay careful attention to the specification when setting questions for the AS exam. If it is not in the specification, it will not be examined. If it is in the specification, it *could* be examined.

In addition to describing the content of the course (which sometimes provides detail that could earn you marks), the specification gives information about the unit tests and about other skills required — for example, using the experience gained by performing practical activities as a basis for improving physiological and psychological understanding. You also need to develop the skills of interpreting and drawing graphs and diagrams.

In addition to looking at the specification, it would be useful for you to read the examiners' reports and mark schemes from previous Unit 1 tests (these are available from AQA). These documents show the depth of knowledge that examiners are looking for, as well as pointing out common mistakes and providing advice on how to achieve good grades.

Study skills and revision strategies

All students need good study skills to be successful. This section provides advice and guidance on how to study AS physical education, together with some strategies for effective revision.

Organising your notes

PE students often accumulate a large quantity of notes, so it is useful to keep this information in an organised manner. The presentation is important; good notes should be clear and concise. You could try organising your notes under main headings and subheadings, with key points highlighted using capitals, italics or colour. Numbered lists can be useful, as can the presentation of information in table form and simple diagrams. For example:

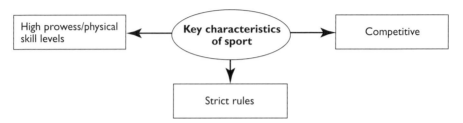

Organising your time

It is a good idea to make a revision timetable to ensure you use your time effectively. This should allow enough time to cover *all* the relevant material. However, it must also be realistic. For many students, revising for longer than an hour at a time becomes counterproductive, so allow for short relaxation breaks or exercise to refresh the body and mind.

Revision strategies

To revise a topic effectively, you should work carefully through your notes, using a copy of the specification to make sure everything is covered. Summarise your notes on the key points in each topic area. Topic cue cards with a summary of key facts and visual representations of the material (e.g. tables, spider diagrams, bubble diagrams) can be useful. These are easily carried around for quick revision. Finally, use the Content Guidance and Questions and Answers sections in this book, discussing any problems or difficulties you have with your teachers or other students.

In many ways you should prepare for a unit test like an athlete prepares for a major event, such as the Olympic Games. An athlete trains every day for weeks or months before the big event, practising the required skills in order to achieve the best result on the day. So it is with exam preparation: everything you do should contribute to your chances of success in the unit test.

The following points summarise some of the strategies that you may wish to use to make sure your revision is as effective as possible:

- Use a revision timetable.
- Ideally, spend time revising in a quiet room, sitting upright at a desk or table, with no distractions.
- Test yourself regularly to assess the effectiveness of your revision. Ask yourself: 'Which techniques work best?' 'What are the gaps in my knowledge?' Remember to revise what you *don't* know.
- Practise past paper questions to highlight gaps in your knowledge and understanding and to improve your technique. You will also become more familiar with the terminology used in exam questions.
- Spend time doing 'active revision', such as:
  — discussing topics with fellow students or teachers
  — summarising your notes
  — compiling revision cue cards
  — answering previous test questions and self-checking against mark schemes

Revision progress

Preparation for exams is a personal thing — you should do what works best for you. You could also draw up, and use, a 'revision progress' table for each topic. An example is shown below.

Complete column 2 to show how you have progressed with your revision:

- N = not revised yet
- P = partly revised
- F = fully revised

Complete column 3 to show how confident you are with the topic:

- 5 = high degree of confidence
- 1 = minimal confidence — the practice questions were poorly answered

The table should be updated as your revision progresses.

Topic: cardiac function	Revised (N/P/F)	Self-evaluation (1–5)
Cardiac cycle		
Cardiac output, stroke volume, heart rate		
Heart rate in response to exercise		
Role of blood carbon dioxide in changing heart rate		
Cardiac hypertrophy		
Starling's law of the heart		
Cardiovascular drift		

It is important to revise every topic, because any area of the specification could appear in the unit test.

The unit test

Unit Test 1 consists of seven *compulsory* questions. There is no choice of question — you have to answer all seven of them. You will have 2 hours to try to earn a maximum of 84 marks, which count for 60% of the total AS marks.

Section A is divided into three sections — applied exercise physiology, skill acquisition and opportunities for participation. There are two questions in each section. Each question is structured and worth 12 marks. Section B comprises one structured question, which is also worth 12 marks. The key difference for the Section B question (Question 7) is that it will be marked according to 'banded statements'. These will include an assessment of the quality of your written communication as well as appropriate subject knowledge. Question 7 is set from the applied anatomy and physiology and applied skill acquisition specification content contained in Unit 2.

It is important to write clearly in the spaces provided within the answer booklet. Avoid writing anything that you want to be marked in the margins because it might not be seen by the examiner if the paper is scanned for online marking.

There are a number of command words and terms commonly used in unit tests. It is important that you understand the meaning of each of these terms and that you answer the question appropriately.

- **Analyse/critically evaluate** — put both sides of an argument or debate, stating your opinions as appropriate.
- **Apply/demonstrate knowledge** — use practical sporting examples to illustrate clearly your understanding of theoretical content.
- **Benefits** — positive outcomes.
- **Characteristics** — features or key distinguishing qualities.
- **Define** — give a clear, concise statement, outlining what is meant by a particular term.
- **Describe** — provide an accurate account of the main points in relation to the task set.
- **Explain** — give reasons to justify statements and opinions given in your answer.
- **State/give/list/identify** — show clear understanding of key characteristics.

Whatever the question style, you must read the wording carefully, underline or highlight key words or phrases, think about your response and allocate time according to the number of marks available. Further advice and guidance on answering Unit 1 questions is provided in the Questions and Answers section of this book.

Content Guidance

Unit 1 is divided into three main topic areas:

- applied exercise physiology
- skill acquisition
- opportunities for participation

In the examination, each topic area has two questions and all questions must be answered.

In addition, Unit 2 contains two elements that you need to be aware of for the Unit 1 exam. Question 7 links to practical scenarios:

- applied exercise physiology in practical situations
- skill acquisition in practical situations

This Content Guidance section summarises the key information that you need to understand and apply in the Unit 1 exam. It also includes useful examiner's tips and hints on 'What the examiner will expect you to be able to do'.

Remember that this Content Guidance is designed to support your revision and should be used in conjunction with your textbook, your own revision notes and other resources.

Applied exercise physiology
Health, exercise and fitness

Definitions of fitness and health

Fitness can be difficult to define because it means different things to different people. One generic definition of fitness is: the ability to perform daily tasks without undue fatigue.

These daily tasks will be quite different for a non-athletic person compared with an elite performer. The fitness requirements of physical activities also vary. For example, the 100 metres sprint requires the body to work anaerobically with great strength, speed and power, whereas the marathon requires good muscular endurance and excellent aerobic capacity.

Health is often defined as: a state of complete physical, mental and social wellbeing, and not merely the absence of disease or infirmity.

Components of fitness

- Components of health-related fitness include cardiorespiratory endurance (also called stamina, VO_2(max) or aerobic capacity), muscular endurance, maximum strength, speed, power and flexibility.
- Components of skill-related fitness include reaction time, coordination and balance.

Definitions of the components of fitness and the methods of testing are given in the following tables.

Health-related components

Component	Definition	Method of testing
Cardiorespiratory endurance (stamina)	The ability to take in and use oxygen during prolonged exercise to delay the onset of fatigue	• Douglas bag • Multistage fitness test • Step test
Muscular endurance	The ability of a muscle to perform repeated contractions and withstand fatigue	NCF abdominal curl
Maximum strength	The maximum force a muscle can exert in a single voluntary contraction	Hand-grip dynamometer
Speed	How fast a person can move a specified distance or how quickly a body part can be put into motion	30 metre sprint test
Power	The amount of work performed per unit of time. It is the product of strength and speed	Vertical jump
Static flexibility	Range of movement round a joint	Sit-and-reach test
Dynamic flexibility	Resistance of a joint to movement	Shoulder flexibility test

Skill-related components

Component	Definition	Method of testing
Reaction time	The time taken from detection of a stimulus to the initiation of a response	Metre ruler test
Agility	Ability to move and position the body quickly and effectively while under control	Illinois agility run
Coordination	The ability of the motor and nervous systems to interact so that motor tasks can be performed more accurately	Alternate hand/wall ball toss
Balance	The ability to keep the centre of mass over the base of support. It can be static, such as a handstand, or dynamic, where balance is retained in motion	Balance board

Effect of lifestyle choices on health and fitness

Individuals make choices in life and these can have an effect on both health and fitness. For example, a poor diet can lead to obesity and health complications. Smoking can affect the efficiency of oxygen transport, and a lack of exercise can lead to heart and mobility problems.

What the examiner will expect you to be able to do
- Give accurate definitions of terms — there might be 2 marks for a definition.

Nutrition

The seven classes of food

Carbohydrates
Simple carbohydrates are found in fruits and are easily digested by the body. They are also present in many processed foods and anything with refined sugar added. **Complex carbohydrates** are found in nearly all plant-based foods, and usually take longer for the body to digest. They are most commonly found in bread, pasta, rice and vegetables.

Carbohydrate is an important source of energy during activity, and it is the main source of energy during high-intensity exercise. Carbohydrates are stored in the muscle and liver as glycogen and transported in the form of glucose. They store a lot of energy and should be consumed before, during and after exercise.

It is important to consider the glycaemic index (release rate) of different carbohydrates and the consequence this has on *when* they should be consumed in relation to training. Foods with a low glycaemic index cause a slow, sustained release of glucose to the blood, whereas foods with a high glycaemic index cause a rapid, sharp rise in blood glucose. Suitable foods to eat 3–4 hours before exercise include beans on toast, pasta or rice with a vegetable-based sauce, breakfast cereal with milk, or crumpets with jam or honey. Suitable snacks to eat 1–2 hours before exercise include fruit smoothies, cereal bars, fruit-flavoured yoghurt and fruit. An hour before exercise, liquid consumption appears to be more important — for example, sports drinks and cordials.

Fats

Fats are the secondary energy fuel for low-intensity aerobic work such as jogging and are made from glycerol and fatty acids. Each glycerol molecule is attached to three fatty acid molecules. Glycerol and fatty acids contain the elements carbon, hydrogen and oxygen. Fats contain a high proportion of carbon, which is why they give us so much energy. Fats are stored in the muscle as triglycerides and transported as fatty acids.

Proteins

Proteins consist of chains of amino acids. They are important for tissue growth and repair and to make enzymes, hormones and haemoglobin. Proteins in the muscles may start to be broken down to provide energy when glycogen and fat stores are low, such as during strenuous activities or sustained periods of exercise.

Vitamins

Vitamins are needed for muscle and nerve functioning, tissue growth and the release of energy from foods. Vitamins cannot be stored in the body and excess amounts are excreted through urine.

Minerals

Minerals assist in bodily functions. For example, calcium is important for strong bones and teeth, and iron helps form haemoglobin, which is needed for the transport of oxygen and therefore to improve stamina levels. Minerals tend to be dissolved by the body as ions and are called electrolytes. These facilitate the transmission of nerve impulses and enable effective muscle contraction, both of which are important during exercise. However, it is important to get the right balance — too much sodium (contained in salt) can result in high blood pressure. As with vitamins, excessive consumption is unlikely to enhance performance.

Fibre

Good sources of fibre are wholemeal bread and pasta, potatoes, nuts, seeds, fruit, vegetables and pulses. Fibre is important during exercise as it can slow down the time it takes the body to break down food, which results in a slower, more sustained, release of energy.

Water

Water constitutes up to 60% of a person's body weight and is essential for good health. It carries nutrients to cells in the body and removes waste products. It also helps to control body temperature. When an athlete starts to exercise, production of water increases (water is a by-product of the aerobic system). We also lose a lot of water through sweat. The volume of water lost depends on the external temperature, the intensity and duration of the exercise and the volume of water consumed before, during and after exercise. Water is important to maintain optimal performance. Sports drinks such as Lucozade Sport and Gatorade can boost glucose levels before and after competition, while water rehydrates during competition.

A balanced diet

A balanced diet should contain 15% protein, 30% fat and 55% carbohydrate. For athletes in training, the percentage of carbohydrate should be increased. Sports nutritionists recommend:
- 10–15% proteins
- 20–25% fats
- 60–75% carbohydrates

The energy balance of food

Energy is obtained from the food we eat (or from what the body stores). It is measured in calories. A calorie (cal) is the amount of heat energy required to raise the temperature of 1 g of water by 1°C. A kilocalorie (kcal) is the amount of heat required to raise the temperature of 1000 g of water by 1°C.

The basic energy requirement of an average person is generally given as 1.3 kcal per hour per kilogram of body weight. So someone who weighs 60 kg requires 1.3 × 24 (hours in a day) × 60 = 1872 kcal per day.

The energy requirement increases during exercise to 8.5 kcal per hour for each kilogram of body weight. So in a 1-hour training session the performer needs an extra 8.5 × 1 × 60 = 510 kcal. The total daily energy requirement of this performer is therefore 1872 + 510 = 2382 kcal.

What should you eat before a competition?

A pre-competition meal should be eaten 3–4 hours before competing because the food needs to be digested and absorbed in order to be useful. The meal needs to be high in carbohydrate, low in fat and moderate in fibre, to aid digestion (foods high in fat, protein and fibre tend to take longer to digest). High levels of carbohydrate will keep the blood glucose levels high throughout the competition/ performance.

Diet of an endurance athlete versus a power athlete

The body's preferred fuel for endurance sport is muscle glycogen. If glycogen stores become depleted, the athlete becomes fatigued and unable to maintain the intensity of training. To replenish and maintain glycogen stores, endurance athletes need a diet rich in carbohydrates — at least 6–10 grams of carbohydrate per kilogram of body weight per day. Water is also essential, to avoid dehydration.

Some endurance athletes manipulate their diet to maximise aerobic energy production. One method is **glycogen loading**, which is covered at A2.

Endurance athletes require more carbohydrates and fats than power athletes because they exercise for longer periods of time and need more energy. Proteins are very important for power athletes. Insufficient protein leads to muscle breakdown. Proteins are necessary for tissue growth and repair.

Body fat composition

This is the physiological make-up of an individual in terms of the distribution of lean body mass and body fat. On average, men have less body fat (15%) than women (25%).

Less body fat generally means a better performance. However, some sports have specific requirements for large amounts of fat, for example the defensive linesman in American football and sumo wrestlers.

Body mass index (BMI)

Body mass index (BMI) takes into account body composition. To calculate BMI, a person's weight in kilograms is divided by his/her height (in metres) squared. For example, a person who is 1.80 m tall weighing 75 kg has a BMI of $75/(1.8 \times 1.8) = 23.15$.

BMI classifications vary but the following is representative of most literature:
- **BMI >19**   underweight
- **BMI 19–25** normal
- **BMI 26–30** overweight
- **BMI 30–40** obese
- **BMI >40**   morbidly obese

Obesity and limitations of definition

Obesity is an excess proportion of total body fat, usually due to energy intake being greater than energy output. Obesity carries an increased risk of heart disease, hypertension, high blood cholesterol, stroke and diabetes. It increases stress on joints and limits flexibility.

An individual is considered to be obese when his/her body weight is 20% or more above normal weight, or when a male accumulates 25% and a female 35% total body fat. The body mass index can also be used as a measure of obesity. An individual is considered obese when his/her BMI is over 30.

What the examiner will expect you to be able to do
- List the seven classes of food and understand the exercise-related function of each food type.
- Compare the dietary requirements of different types of athlete.
- Identify what is meant by obesity, body mass index and body fat composition and link these to diet.

Pulmonary function

The mechanics of breathing

Air moves from areas of high pressure to areas of low pressure. The greater the pressure difference, the faster air flows.

Changing the volume of the thoracic cavity alters the pressure of air in the lungs. **Inspiration** increases the volume of the thoracic cavity through contraction of the muscles surrounding the lungs. This reduces the pressure of air in the lungs. **Expiration** decreases the volume of the thoracic cavity. This increases the pressure of air in the lungs, forcing air out. At rest, expiration is a passive process.

Respiratory muscles

Ventilation phase	Muscles used during breathing at rest	Muscles used during exercise
Inspiration	Diaphragm	Diaphragm
	External intercostals	• External intercostals • Sternocleidomastoid • Scalenes • Pectoralis major
Expiration	Diaphragm and external intercostals relax (passive process)	• Internal intercostals • Abdominals

Respiratory volumes

Definitions and values of respiratory volumes, and the way they change during exercise, are given in the table below.

Lung volume or capacity	Definition	Average values at rest (litres)	Change during exercise
Tidal volume	Volume of air breathed in or out per breath	0.5	Increase
Inspiratory reserve volume	Volume of air that can be forcibly inspired after a normal breath	3.1	Decrease
Expiratory reserve volume	Volume of air that can be forcibly expired after a normal breath	1.2	Slight decrease
Residual volume	Volume of air that remains in the lungs after maximum expiration	1.2	No change
Vital capacity	Volume of air forcibly expired after maximum inspiration in one breath	4.8	No change
Minute ventilation	Volume of air breathed in or out per minute	6	Large increase
Total lung capacity	Vital capacity + residual volume	6	No change

Lung capacities can be measured from a spirometer trace.

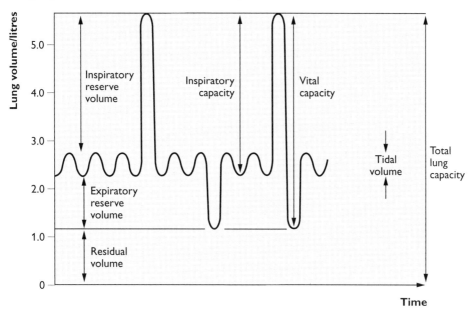

Gaseous exchange at the lungs

Gaseous exchange at the lungs is concerned with the replenishment of oxygen in the blood and the removal of carbon dioxide.

Diffusion is the movement of a gas from an area of high concentration to an area of low concentration down a concentration gradient until equilibrium is reached. In the lungs, diffusion of gases is aided by the structure of the alveoli. Alveoli are only one cell thick, so there is a short diffusion pathway; they have a vast surface area, which facilitates diffusion; and they are surrounded by a dense network of capillaries. The rate of diffusion is approximately 250 cm^3 of oxygen per minute at rest but this can rise to over 5 litres of oxygen per minute during exercise.

Oxygen makes up approximately 21% of air, so it exerts a **partial pressure**. Gases flow from areas of high pressure to areas of low pressure. As oxygen moves from the alveoli to the blood and then to the muscle, its partial pressure in each has to be successively lower.

The exchange of gases in the lungs takes place between alveolar air and blood flowing through the lung (pulmonary) capillaries. Oxygen enters the blood from the alveoli because the partial pressure of oxygen in the alveoli (105 mmHg) is higher than the partial pressure of oxygen in the incoming blood vessels (40 mmHg). This is because the working muscles remove oxygen, so its concentration in the blood is lower and therefore so is its partial pressure. The difference between any two pressures is referred to as the pressure gradient and the steeper this gradient, the faster diffusion will be. Oxygen diffuses from the alveoli into the blood until the pressure is equal in both.

The movement of carbon dioxide occurs similarly but from the blood to the alveoli, because the partial pressure of carbon dioxide in the blood is higher (46 mmHg) than that in the alveoli (40 mmHg).

Inspired air contains more oxygen than expired air; expired air contains more carbon dioxide than inspired air. The percentage concentrations of gases found in inspired and expired air are shown in the table below.

	Inspired air (%)	Expired air at rest (%)	Expired air during exercise (%)
Oxygen	21	16.4	15
Carbon dioxide	0.03	4.0	6

Gaseous exchange at the tissues

This takes place between arterial blood, flowing through the tissue capillaries, and the cells. Oxygen diffuses out of the arterial blood and into the muscle cells because the partial pressure of oxygen is higher (100 mmHg) in the blood than in the cells (40 mmHg).

Arterio-venous difference

This is the difference between the oxygen content of the arterial blood arriving at the muscles and the venous blood leaving the muscles. At rest, the arterio-venous difference is low because the muscles do not require much oxygen. However, during exercise the muscles need more oxygen, so the arterio-venous difference is high. This increase in A-VO$_2$ affects gaseous exchange at the alveoli. There is a higher concentration of carbon dioxide and a lower level of oxygen in the venous blood returning to the heart (and then being sent to the lungs). This increases the diffusion gradient of both gases.

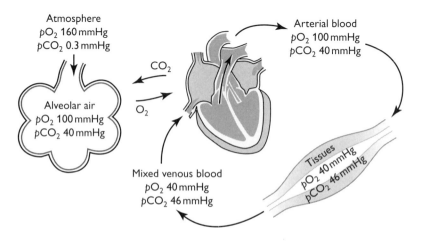

Training also increases the arterio-venous difference, because trained performers can extract more oxygen from the blood.

The diagram on page 18 highlights the differences in the partial pressure of oxygen and carbon dioxide in the alveoli, blood and muscle cells, and shows the A-VO$_2$ difference.

Transport of oxygen

Only about 3% of oxygen dissolves in plasma; 97% combines with **haemoglobin** to form **oxyhaemoglobin**. When fully saturated, each haemoglobin molecule carries four oxygen molecules. At the tissues, oxygen dissociates from haemoglobin because of the lower pressure of oxygen in the tissues. In the muscle cells, oxygen is taken up by myoglobin. This has a high affinity for oxygen, which means that it can act as an oxygen store. During exercise, there is increased cellular respiration. As a result, the partial pressure of oxygen in the cell decreases to the point where myoglobin gives up its oxygen to the mitochondria.

The relationship of oxygen and haemoglobin can be represented by the oxyhaemoglobin dissociation curve.

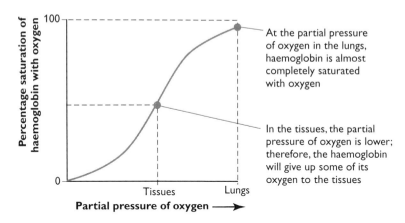

During exercise, there is an increased demand for oxygen. Exercise creates conditions that cause haemoglobin to release some of its oxygen more readily. These conditions are:
- an increase in temperature in the blood and muscle
- a decrease in the partial pressure of oxygen in the muscle, which increases the oxygen diffusion gradient
- an increase in carbon dioxide in the muscle, which increases the carbon dioxide diffusion gradient
- an increase in acidity (lower pH), which causes oxygen to dissociate from haemoglobin more quickly (Bohr effect, see the following diagram)

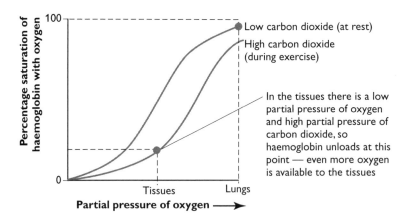

Control of ventilation

The nervous system can increase or decrease the rate, depth and rhythm of breathing. The control of ventilation is summarised in the diagram below.

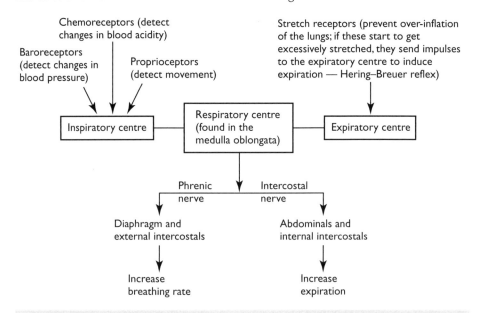

What the examiner will expect you to be able to do

- Describe the mechanics of breathing at rest and during exercise.
- Identify the different lung volumes and label them on a spirometer trace.
- Describe gaseous exchange at the alveoli and the muscles.
- Explain the principles of diffusion and the importance of partial pressures.
- Explain and label the oxyhaemoglobin dissociation curve.
- Explain how breathing is controlled.

The vascular system: transport of blood gases

Circulation

There are two types of circulation:

- **pulmonary** circulation takes deoxygenated blood from the heart to the lungs and returns oxygenated blood from the lungs to the heart
- **systemic** circulation carries oxygenated blood from the heart to the body tissues and returns deoxygenated blood from the body tissues to the heart

Blood vessels

The vascular system consists of five different types of blood vessel that carry the blood from the heart, distribute it around the body and return it to the heart.

Arteries carry blood away from the heart. Each heartbeat pushes blood through the arteries by a surge of pressure. The elastic arterial walls expand with each surge, which can be felt as a pulse in the arteries near the surface of the skin. The arteries then branch off and divide into smaller vessels called **arterioles**, which in turn divide into microscopic vessels called **capillaries**. A capillary wall consists of a single layer of endothelium cells. Capillaries are only wide enough to allow red blood cells to pass through one at a time. The exchange of substances with the tissues takes place across the capillary walls and the blood then flows from the capillaries to the **venules**, which gradually increase in size and eventually form **veins**. To summarise, the order in which the blood flows through the vascular system is:

heart ⟶ arteries ⟶ arterioles ⟶ capillaries ⟶ venules ⟶ veins ⟶ heart

The important features of arteries, capillaries and veins are summarised in the table below.

Feature	Artery	Capillary	Vein
Tunica externa — outer layer containing collagen fibres	Present	Absent	Present
Tunica media — middle layer made up of elastic fibres and smooth muscle	Thick with many elastic fibres	Absent	Thinner and less elastic than in an artery
Tunica interna — inner layer made up of thin epithelial cells that are smooth to reduce friction	Present	Present	Present
Size of lumen	Small	Microscopic	Large
Valves	Absent	Absent	Present

The pulse

The pulse is a wave of pressure generated when the left ventricle pumps blood into the aorta, which is the main artery. The pulse can be felt at a number of places in the body — the radial artery in the wrist and the carotid artery in the neck are the two most common sites. Other sites include the femoral, brachial and temporal arteries.

Venous return

This is the term used for blood that is returned to the right side of the heart through the veins. Up to 70% of the total blood volume is contained in the veins at rest. This provides a large reservoir of blood that can be returned rapidly to the heart when needed.

The heart can only pump out as much blood as it receives, so cardiac output is dependent on venous return. A rapid increase in venous return enables a significant increase in stroke volume and therefore cardiac output. Veins have a large lumen and offer little resistance to blood flow. By the time blood enters the veins, blood pressure is low. This means that active mechanisms are needed to ensure venous return:

- **Skeletal muscle pump** — when muscles contract and relax, they change shape so that the muscles press on nearby veins, causing a pumping effect and squeezing the blood towards the heart.
- **Respiratory pump** — when muscles contract and relax during inspiration and expiration, pressure changes occur in the thoracic and abdominal cavities, compressing the nearby veins and enabling blood to return to the heart.
- **Valves** — ensure that blood in the veins flows in only one direction: once the blood has passed through a valve, the valve closes to prevent the blood from flowing back.
- **Smooth muscle** — a thin layer of smooth muscle in the walls of the veins helps to squeeze blood back towards the heart.

Oxygen and carbon dioxide in the vascular system

Oxygen plays a major role in energy production. A reduction in the amount of oxygen in the body has a detrimental impact on performance. During exercise, when oxygen diffuses into the capillaries supplying the skeletal muscles, 3% dissolves in plasma and 97% combines with haemoglobin to form oxyhaemoglobin. At the tissues, oxygen dissociates from haemoglobin because of the lower pressure of oxygen that exists there. In the muscle, oxygen is stored by **myoglobin**. This has a high affinity for oxygen and stores the oxygen until it can be transported from the capillaries to the mitochondria. The mitochondria are the sites in the muscle where aerobic respiration takes place.

Carbon dioxide is transported around the body in the following ways:

- 70% is transported in the blood as hydrogen carbonate (bicarbonate) ions. The carbon dioxide produced by the muscles as a waste product diffuses into the bloodstream, where it combines with water to form carbonic acid. Carbonic acid is a weak acid that dissociates into hydrogen carbonate ions.
- 23% combines with haemoglobin to form carbaminohaemoglobin.
- 7% dissolves in plasma.

An increase in the level of carbon dioxide results in an increase in blood and tissue acidity. This is detected by chemoreceptors, which send impulses to the medulla. Heart rate, breathing rate and transport increase so that more carbon dioxide is exhaled and the arterial blood levels of both oxygen and carbon dioxide are maintained.

Blood pressure

Blood pressure is the force exerted by the blood against the blood vessel wall. It is measured at the brachial artery (in the upper arm) using a sphygmomanometer. A typical reading at rest is 120/80 mmHg (millimetres of mercury).

Blood pressure varies in the different types of blood vessel and is largely dependent on the distance of the blood vessel from the heart:
- arteries — high and in pulses
- arterioles — not quite as high as in arteries
- capillaries — pressure drops throughout the capillary network
- veins — low

Blood velocity

The velocity of blood flow depends on the total cross-sectional area of the blood vessel. The smaller the cross-sectional area, the faster the blood flows. Although the capillaries are the smallest of the blood vessels, the fact that there are so many of them means that the total cross-sectional area is much greater than that of the arteries. This means that the flow of blood is slower in the capillaries and this allows enough time for efficient exchange of substances with the tissues. The relationship between blood velocity and cross-sectional area of the different blood vessels is shown in the diagram below.

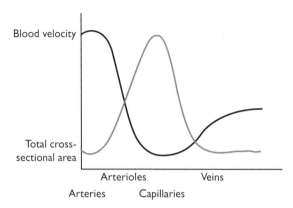

Effects of exercise on blood pressure and blood volume

During aerobic exercise, systolic pressure increases due to an increase in cardiac output. Diastolic pressure remains constant. During isometric work, diastolic pressure also increases due to increased resistance in the blood vessels.

A decrease in blood volume occurs during exercise when plasma moves out of the capillaries and into the surrounding tissues. After a period of training, blood volume increases, due mainly to an increase in the volume of blood plasma and a small increase in the number of red blood cells.

Vasomotor control

The **vasomotor centre** is located in the medulla oblongata of the brain. It controls both blood pressure and blood flow. During exercise, chemical changes are detected by chemoreceptors while higher blood pressure is detected by baroreceptors. These receptors stimulate the vasomotor centre, which redistributes blood flow by vasodilation and vasoconstriction:
- vasodilation increases blood flow
- vasoconstriction decreases blood flow

The vascular shunt

During exercise, the working muscles need more oxygen, so vasodilation occurs in the arterioles supplying the skeletal muscles, increasing blood flow and bringing in the much-needed oxygen. At the same time, vasoconstriction occurs in the arterioles supplying other organs, such as the intestines and the liver. This redirection of blood flow is known as shunting, or the **vascular shunt** mechanism.

Precapillary sphincters also aid blood redistribution. These are tiny rings of muscle located at the opening of capillaries. When they contract, blood flow is restricted through the capillary and when they relax, blood flow is increased. During exercise, the precapillary sphincters of the capillary networks supplying skeletal muscle relax. This increases blood flow, which in turn helps to saturate the tissues with oxygen.

Blood flow to the brain remains constant to ensure that brain function is maintained.

> **What the examiner will expect you to be able to do**
> - Identify the changes in blood flow during exercise and explain how they occur through vasoconstriction and vasodilation. Questions on the vascular shunt mechanism occur frequently.

Cardiac function

The cardiac cycle

The diastole phase is when the chambers of the heart are relaxing and filling with blood. The systole phase is when the heart contracts and forces blood either around the heart or out of the heart to the lungs and the body. The diastole phase lasts for about 0.5 seconds; the systole phase lasts for 0.3 seconds. The cardiac cycle is summarised in the following table.

Stage	Action	Result
Atrial systole	Atrial walls contract	Blood is forced through the bicuspid and tricuspid valves into the ventricles
Atrial diastole	Atrial walls relax	Blood enters the right atrium via the vena cava and the left atrium via the pulmonary vein but cannot pass into the ventricles, because the tricuspid and bicuspid valves are closed
Ventricular systole	Ventricular walls contract	Pressure of blood opens the semilunar valves and blood is ejected into the pulmonary artery and the aorta. The tricuspid and bicuspid valves close
Ventricular diastole	Ventricular walls relax	Blood enters from the atria (passive ventricular filling, *not* due to atrial contraction). The semilunar valves are closed

The cardiac cycle is triggered by an electrical impulse called the cardiac impulse or the conduction system.

The conduction system

When the heart beats, blood flows through it in a controlled manner — in through the atria and out through the ventricles. Heart muscle is described as **myogenic** because the beat starts in the heart muscle itself, with an electrical signal in the sino-atrial node (pacemaker). This electrical signal then spreads through the heart in what is often described as a wave of excitation.

From the sinoatrial node, the electrical signal spreads through the walls of the atria, causing them to contract and force blood into the ventricles. The signal then passes through the atrioventricular node in the atrioventricular septum. This delays the transmission of the cardiac impulse for approximately 0.1 seconds to enable the atria to contract fully before ventricular contraction begins. The electrical signal then passes down through specialised fibres called the bundle of His. This is located in the septum separating the two ventricles. The bundle of His branches into two bundle branches and then moves into smaller bundles called Purkyne fibres, which spread throughout the ventricles. When the impulse passes through these fibres, it causes them to contract.

Cardiac terms

Stroke volume

This is the amount of blood pumped out by the left ventricle in each contraction. The average resting stroke volume is approximately 70 ml. Stroke volume is determined by:

- Venous return — the volume of blood returning to the heart through the veins. If venous return increases, stroke volume will also increase (i.e. if more blood enters the heart, more blood is pumped out).

- The elasticity of cardiac fibres — the volume of blood in the ventricle increases during diastole and stretches the cardiac fibres. The more they stretch, the greater the force of contraction, which increases stroke volume. This is called **Starling's law.**
- The contractility of the cardiac tissue (myocardium) — the greater the contractility of cardiac tissue, the greater the force of contraction. This results in an increase in stroke volume.
- An increase in the ejection fraction (the percentage of blood pumped out by the left ventricle per beat). An average value is 60% but it can increase by up to 85% following a period of training.

Heart rate

This is the number of times the heart beats per minute. The average resting heart rate is approximately 72 beats per minute.

Cardiac output

This is the amount of blood pumped out by *each* ventricle per minute. It is equal to stroke volume multiplied by heart rate:

$$\text{cardiac output } (Q) = \text{stroke volume} \times \text{heart rate}$$
$$Q = 70 \times 72$$
$$= 5\,040 \text{ ml } (5.04 \text{ litres})$$

Cardiac output and exercise

Regular aerobic training results in hypertrophy of the cardiac muscle — the heart muscle gets bigger. This has important effects on stroke volume and heart rate, and therefore on cardiac output. A bigger heart enables more blood to be pumped out per beat (i.e. stroke volume increases). In more complex language, the end diastolic volume of the ventricle increases. If the ventricle can contract with more force and push out more blood, the heart does not have to beat so often. Therefore, the resting heart rate decreases. This is called **bradycardia**. The increase in stroke volume and decrease in resting heart rate mean that cardiac output at rest remains unchanged. However, during exercise an increase in heart rate, coupled with an increase in stroke volume, results in an increase in cardiac output.

The following table shows the differences in cardiac output (to the nearest litre) in a trained and an untrained individual at rest and during exercise. The individuals are aged 18 so their maximum heart rate is 202 beats per minute. (A person's maximum heart rate is calculated as 220 minus his/her age.)

Condition	Stroke volume/cm³	Heart rate/bpm	Q/litres
Untrained, at rest	70	72	5
Untrained, during exercise	120	202	24
Trained, at rest	85	60	5
Trained, during exercise	170	202	34

This increase in cardiac output has huge benefits for trained individuals. It means that more blood, and therefore more oxygen, is delivered to the working muscles. In addition, when the body starts to exercise, the distribution of blood flow changes — a higher proportion of blood passes to the working muscles and less goes to other organs such as the intestine.

Stroke volume in response to exercise

Stroke volume increases with exercise intensity but only up to 40–60% of maximum effort, at which point it levels out. One explanation is that the increased heart rate at near maximum effort results in a shorter diastolic phase. The ventricles have less time to fill with blood, so they cannot pump as much out.

Heart rate range in response to exercise

The heart rate response to maximal and submaximal exercise and during recovery from exercise is shown on the graphs below.

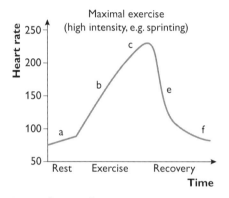 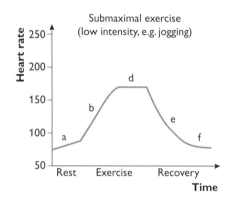

Key to the graphs:

a = **anticipatory rise** due to the action of the hormone adrenaline, which makes the heart beat faster and stronger

b = sharp rise in heart rate at the beginning of exercise, mainly due to anaerobic work

c = heart rate continuing to rise due to maximal workloads stressing the anaerobic system

d = steady state as the athlete is able to meet the oxygen demand for the activity

e = rapid decline in heart rate as soon as the exercise stops, owing to a decrease in the demand for oxygen by the working muscles

f = slow recovery as the body systems return to resting levels (but the heart rate stays elevated to rid the body of waste products such as lactic acid)

Control of heart rate

Heart rate increases during exercise to ensure that the working muscles receive more oxygen. The heart generates its own impulses from the sinoatrial node but the rate at which these impulses are fired is controlled by two main mechanisms — neural and hormonal.

Neural control involves the autonomic nervous system, which comprises the sympathetic system and the parasympathetic system. The sympathetic system stimulates the heart to beat faster; the parasympathetic system returns the heart rate to its resting level. The cardiac control centre located in the medulla oblongata of the brain co-ordinates these two systems.

The cardiac control centre is stimulated by:
- chemoreceptors — which detect increases in carbon dioxide and lactic acid and decreases in oxygen
- baroreceptors — which detect increases in blood pressure
- proprioceptors — which detect increases in muscle movement

The cardiac control centre then sends an impulse through the sympathetic nervous system or the cardiac accelerator nerve to the sinoatrial node and heart rate increases.

The **hormonal control mechanism** involves adrenaline and noradrenaline. These are stress hormones released by the adrenal glands. Exercise causes a stress-induced adrenaline response. This results in:
- stimulation of the sinoatrial node, which results in an increase in both the speed and force of contraction
- an increase in blood pressure due to the constriction of blood vessels
- an increase in blood glucose levels — glucose is used by the muscles for energy

Cardiovascular drift

It used to be thought that exercising at a steady level led to the body reaching a steady state where the heart rate remained constant. However, new research has shown that heart rate increases slowly. This is called **cardiovascular drift**. Cardiovascular drift is characterised by a progressive decrease in stroke volume and arterial blood pressure, together with the progressive rise in heart rate. It occurs during prolonged exercise in a warm environment despite the intensity of the exercise remaining the same. It is suggested that cardiovascular drift occurs because a portion of the fluid volume lost when we sweat comes from the plasma volume. The decrease in plasma volume reduces venous return and stroke volume. Heart rate increases to compensate and maintain constant cardiac output. To minimise cardiovascular drift, it is important to maintain high fluid consumption before and during prolonged exercise.

Effects of training on the heart

Physiological adaptations take place after a period of training and these will make the initial training sessions appear very easy. This is because more oxygen can be taken in, transported and utilised by the muscle cells.

The effects of training on cardiac function include **athlete's heart**, which is the common term for an enlarged heart caused by repeated strenuous exercise. Due to the increased demands of exercise, the chambers of the heart enlarge, as does muscle mass (**hypertrophy**). This results in an increase in the volume of blood that can be pumped out per beat, i.e. a rise in stroke volume and maximum cardiac output. Consequently, the heart has to contract less frequently and there is a decrease in resting heart rate (**bradycardia**).

Increased capillarisation of the heart muscle increases the efficiency of oxygen diffusion into the myocardium. Resistance or strength training causes an increase in the force of heart contractions due to a thickening of the ventricular myocardium. This increases stroke volume and ejection fraction, as a higher percentage of blood is pumped.

> **What the examiner will expect you to be able to do**
> - Identify the stages of the cardiac cycle and link them to the conduction system.
> - Define the terms cardiac output, stroke volume and heart rate, and explain both the changes that occur during exercise and how these changes come about.
> - Explain the term cardiovascular drift.
> - Describe how heart rate is controlled.
> - Explain the effects of training on the heart.

Analysis of movement

Axes and planes of the body

To help explain movement, the body can be pictured as having a series of imaginary slices running through it. These are called **planes of movement**. They divide the body in three ways:
- The **sagittal** plane is a vertical plane that divides the body into right and left sides.
- The **frontal** (coronal) plane is also a vertical plane but this divides the body into front and back.
- The **transverse** plane is a horizontal plane that divides the body into upper and lower parts.

The body (or body parts) moves in one or more of these planes, depending on the action being performed. In a full twisting somersault, for example, the gymnast moves in all three planes.

There are three **axes of movement**:
- The transverse axis runs from side to side across the body.
- The sagittal axis runs from front to back.
- The vertical axis runs from top to bottom.

Most movements occurring at joints are related to both axes and planes. For example, flexion and extension occur in a sagittal plane about a transverse axis; rotation occurs in a transverse plane about a vertical axis; abduction and adduction occur in a frontal plane about a sagittal axis.

Analysis of movement

You are expected to know the muscles and bones involved in the following movements:

- the shoulder and elbow actions in push-ups, over-arm throwing and forehand racket strokes
- the hip, knee and ankle actions in running, kicking, jumping and squats

These are summarised in the following tables.

Ball-and-socket joints

Joint	Articulating bones	Movement	Agonist
Hip	Acetabulum of the pelvis and femur	Flexion	Iliopsoas (hip flexors)
		Extension	Gluteus maximus
		Lateral (outward) rotation	Gluteus maximus
		Medial (inward) rotation	Gluteus minimus
		Abduction	Gluteus maximus
		Adduction	Adductors (longus, brevis and magnus)
Shoulder	Glenoid fossa of the scapula and humerus	Flexion	Anterior deltoid
		Extension	Latissimus dorsi
		Lateral (outward) rotation	Infraspinatus
		Medial (inward) rotation	Subscapularis
		Abduction	Middle deltoid
		Adduction	Pectoralis major
		Horizontal flexion	Pectoralis major
		Horizontal extension	Latissimus dorsi

Hinge joints

Joint	Articulating bones	Movement	Agonist
Elbow	Radius, ulna and humerus	Flexion	Biceps brachii
		Extension	Triceps brachii
Knee	Tibia and femur	Flexion	Hamstrings
		Extension	Quadriceps
Ankle	Tibia, fibula and talus	Plantarflexion	Gastrocnemius
		Dorsiflexion	Tibialis anterior

Practical examples

Right leg action in kicking
- Hip joint — flexion
  - Agonist: hip flexors (iliopsoas)
  - Antagonist: gluteus maximus
- Knee joint — extension
  - Agonist: quadriceps (rectus femoris)
  - Antagonist: hamstrings (biceps femoris)

Leg action in squats (downward phase)
- Hip joint — flexion
  - Agonist: gluteals
  - Antagonist: iliopsoas
- Knee joint — flexion
  - Agonist: quadriceps
  - Antagonist: hamstrings

In these two joints the agonist and antagonist appear to be the wrong way round. This is because an eccentric contraction is being performed.

Right shoulder and arm actions during the beginning of the tennis serve
- Shoulder — abduction
  - Agonist: deltoid (middle)
  - Antagonist: latissimus dorsi
- Elbow joint — flexion
  - Agonist: biceps brachii
  - Antagonist: triceps brachii

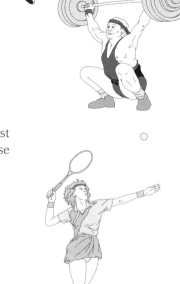

Types of muscular contraction

A muscle can contract in three different ways, depending on the muscle action that is required.

Concentric contraction
The muscle shortens under tension — for example, during the upward phase of an arm curl, the biceps brachii performs a concentric contraction as it shortens to produce flexion of the elbow.

Eccentric contraction
The muscle lengthens under tension (and does not relax). When a muscle contracts eccentrically it is acting as a brake to help control the movement of the body part during negative work. For example, when landing from a standing jump, the quadriceps muscles are performing negative work as they are supporting the weight of the

body during landing. The knee joint is in the flexed position but the quadriceps muscles are unable to relax, as the weight of the body ensures that they lengthen under tension.

Isometric contraction
The muscle contracts without lengthening or shortening. The result is that no movement occurs. An isometric contraction occurs when a muscle acts as a fixator or against a resistance.

Muscle function

A muscle can perform three functions:
- **agonist** — the muscle shortens under tension to produce movement
- **antagonist** — the muscle relaxes or lengthens to allow the agonist to shorten
- **fixator** — the muscle increases in tension but no movement occurs. A fixator is normally located at the joint where the origin of the agonist occurs. For example, in the upward phase of an arm curl, the biceps brachii contracts and is the agonist. Its origin is in the shoulder, so the deltoid acts as a fixator during this movement.

Antagonistic muscle action
Using flexion of the elbow as an example, the biceps brachii contracts and is responsible for the movement. It is said to be acting as an agonist or prime mover. An antagonist muscle is one that works in opposition to the agonist. When the biceps brachii is contracting, the triceps brachii is lengthening and acting as the antagonist. When one muscle is acting as an agonist and the other is acting as the antagonist, the muscles are said to be working together as a pair to produce the required movement. This is called **antagonistic muscle action**.

Levers

A lever has three main components:
- a pivot (fulcrum)
- the weight to be moved (resistance)
- a source of energy (effort or force)

In the body, the skeleton forms a system of levers that allows us to move. The bones act as the levers, the joints are the fulcrums and the muscles provide the effort.

The main functions of a lever are:
- to increase the speed at which the body can move
- to increase the resistance that a given effort can move

Classification of levers
There are three types of lever:
- First-order lever — the fulcrum is between the effort and the resistance. First-order levers can increase both the effects of the effort and the speed of the body. An example can be seen in the elbow during extension of the arm.

- Second-order lever — the resistance lies between the fulcrum and the effort. Second-order levers generally increase only the effect of the effort. Plantarflexion of the ankle involves the use of a second-order lever.
- Third-order lever — the effort lies between the fulcrum and the resistance. Third-order levers are responsible for most of the movements of the human body. They can increase the body's ability to move quickly but in terms of applying force they are very inefficient. An example can be seen in the forearm during flexion of the elbow.

The **effort arm** or **force arm** is the shortest perpendicular distance between the fulcrum and the application of force (effort). The **resistance arm** is the shortest perpendicular distance between the fulcrum and the resistance. The diagram below illustrates the force arm and the resistance arm in a third-order lever.

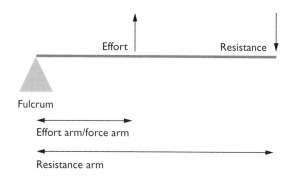

When the resistance arm is longer than the force arm, the lever system is at a **mechanical disadvantage**. This means that it cannot move as heavy a load but it can move the load faster. When the force arm is longer than the resistance arm, the lever system is at a **mechanical advantage**. This means that it can move a large load over a short distance and requires little effort.

What the examiner will expect you to be able to do

- Explain how the body moves in relation to planes and axes during specific exercises. Most of the movements required for AQA involve flexion and extension in the sagittal plane and transverse axis.
- Name the muscles, bones and movements involved in the shoulder and arm action in push-ups, over-arm throwing and forehand racket strokes, and in the hip, knee and ankle action in running, kicking, jumping and squats.
- Apply knowledge of the joints, muscles, movements, types of muscle contraction and muscle function.
- Classify a lever as first, second or third order and relate the lever to effective performance. Most of the levers in the body are third-order, but remember that the ankle is a second-order lever — and frequently appears in exams.

Applied exercise physiology in practical situations

This section will be taught through the practical component of your course (Unit 2). It will be examined as part of the extended question in Section B of the Unit 1 test.

Principles of training

An effective training programme will include the six principles of training:

- **overload** (FITT) — this is achieved by increasing one or more of the following:
  - **frequency** (the number of times that you train per week)
  - **intensity** (how hard you work)
  - **time** (the length of the training session)
  - **type** of training
- **progression** — this involves the gradual application of overload
- **specificity** — the training should be relevant
- **reversibility** — this is often referred to as detraining
- **moderation** — don't overdo it, because over-training can lead to injury
- **variance** — a training programme needs to have variety in order to maintain interest and motivation

Calculating working intensities for optimal gains

Heart rate

Heart rate training zones can be used to gauge how hard you are working. Most training zones are calculated from maximum heart rate, which is calculated as 220 minus age. So if you are 17, your maximum heart rate is 220 − 17 = 203.

You need to work at a certain percentage of your maximum heart rate. The **Karvonen principle** is more accurate than other methods because it takes into account an individual's fitness level by using resting heart rate to work out the training zone. Karvonen suggests a training intensity of 60–75% of maximum heart rate, using the following calculation:

60% = resting heart rate + 0.60 × (maximum heart rate − resting heart rate)

75% = resting heart rate + 0.75 × (maximum heart rate − resting heart rate)

For a 17-year-old with a resting heart rate of 60 beats per minute the calculation is:

60% = 60 + 0.6 (203 − 60)   75% = 60 + 0.75 (203 − 60)
    = 60 + 0.6 × 143   = 60 + 0.75 × 143
    = 60 + 86 = **146**   = 60 + 107 = **167**

So a 17-year-old with a resting heart rate of 60 beats per minute, working at an intensity of 60–75% of maximum heart rate, should be working with a heart rate between 146 and 167 beats per minute.

Borg scale

The Borg scale is a simple method of rating perceived exertion (RPE) and is used to measure a performer's level of intensity during training. Perceived exertion is how hard you feel your body is working. During exercise, the Borg scale is used to assign numbers to how you feel. If you feel you are working too hard, you can reduce the intensity. The most common RPE scales are the 15-point scale and the 9-point scale.

1 rep max (1RM)

When weight training you need to work out your one repetition maximum (1RM) for each exercise, so that you can decide on the intensity that you want to train at. There are different types of strength and you need to decide which type you want to improve. Depending on strength type, you need to work at a certain percentage of your 1RM. For example:
- maximum strength, 85% and over of 1RM
- power (elastic strength), 70–85% of 1RM
- muscular endurance, 50–70% of 1RM

Fitness testing

Fitness testing measures a performer's ability. It can highlight strengths and weaknesses, motivate the performer and progress can be monitored through retesting.

Validity and reliability of testing

When carrying out the various fitness tests, it is important to consider their validity and reliability.

Validity — does the test measure exactly what it sets out to? For example, the 'sit-and-reach' test for flexibility only covers the hamstrings and lower back. Therefore it is a valid test for the lower body but not for the upper body.

Is the test sport specific? It is important to conduct a test that replicates sporting actions and uses the muscles in the same way they are used in the performer's activity. For example, the multistage fitness test involves running, so it is valid for a games player where a lot of running is involved, but less so for a cyclist or a swimmer.

Reliability — is the test accurate? In order for the step test to be reliable, the correct procedure must be maintained, i.e. everyone who completes the test should do so at the same rate, height and cadence and there should be full extension between steps.

When testing, the following factors should be taken into account:
- The tester should be experienced.
- The equipment should be standardised.
- Sequencing of tests is important.
- Performers should be motivated to complete the test to the best of their abilities.
- Tests should be repeated to minimise the effects of human error.

Principles of maximal and submaximal tests

Maximal tests are performed when the athlete is working at maximum effort, usually to exhaustion. The tests are reliable and objective. Examples of anaerobic maximal tests are the 30 metres sprint and the Wingate test. Aerobic maximal tests include the multistage fitness test and Cooper's 12-minute run.

Disadvantages of these types of tests are as follows:
- It is difficult to ensure that the performer is actually working to a maximum.
- It is hard to stay motivated when pushing yourself to exhaustion.
- There are possible dangers of over-exertion and injury.

Submaximal tests are not exhaustive and do not require the performer to work at maximal levels. Aerobic examples of these tests include the Harvard step test and the PWC170 test. Motivation is not an issue but these tests rely on data that are predictive or estimated, and there are problems with accuracy and objectivity.

Warming up and cooling down

The warm-up

Warming up prepares the body for exercise and should be carried out at the start of every training session. The first stage of a warm-up should be light cardiovascular exercise, such as jogging, to gently increase the pulse. This increases cardiac output and breathing rate, and directs more blood to the working muscles via the vascular shunt.

The second stage involves stretching and flexibility exercises, especially with the joints and muscles that will be most active during the training session.

The third stage should include the movement patterns to be carried out — for example practising shooting in basketball and netball, or dribbling in hockey and football.

These three stages together increase the amount of oxygen delivered to the muscles and at the same time reduce the risk of injury.

A warm-up has the following physiological effects:
- The release of adrenaline increases heart rate and dilates the capillaries, allowing more oxygen to be delivered to the working muscles.
- Muscle temperature increases, which enables oxygen to dissociate more easily from haemoglobin and allows for an increase in enzyme activity, making energy readily available.
- The speed of nerve impulse conduction increases, which raises alertness.
- The increase in muscle temperature leads to greater elasticity of the muscle fibres, which increases the speed and force of muscle contraction.
- Efficient movement at joints occurs through an increased production of synovial fluid.

The psychological benefits of a warm-up include:
- it enables the performer to focus on the task in hand
- it reduces anxiety
- it allows mental rehearsal

The cool-down

A cool-down should be performed after any physical activity, as it helps to return the body to its pre-exercise state more quickly.

A cool-down consists of light exercise to keep the heart rate elevated. This keeps blood flow high and allows oxygen to be flushed through the muscles, oxidising and removing any lactic acid that remains. Performing light exercise also allows the skeletal muscle pump to keep working, which maintains venous return and prevents blood from pooling in the veins.

A cool-down may help to limit the effect of DOMS (delayed onset of muscle soreness). DOMS arises from structural damage to muscle fibres and connective tissue surrounding the fibres, usually following excessive eccentric contraction when the muscle fibres are put under a lot of strain.

The psychological value of a cool-down includes:
- it allows the performer to focus on errors before the next game
- it reduces stress

Principles of safe practice

Apart from warming up and cooling down to help prevent injury and muscle soreness following exercise, there are some other factors to consider:
- Which exercises to perform and in what order — e.g. in circuit training the muscle groups should be rotated.
- Dehydration — performers should drink plenty of water during exercise.
- Rest days or recovery periods should be included in training sessions.
- The correct techniques must be used, especially in stretching and weight training.
- Equipment must be safety-checked.
- Athletes training in a cold environment should wear plenty of layers of clothing.
- Sports halls should be clean and free from potential dangers.
- Differences in performance due to gender and age should be considered. Men generally have more strength than women but the opposite can be true for flexibility.
- Training should be progressive, whether you are fully fit or returning from injury.

Training methods

Continuous training

This involves exercise without rest intervals, which places stress on the aerobic energy system. It concentrates on developing endurance. Examples include cycling, jogging and swimming. To make improvements in aerobic fitness, it is important to apply the principles of training (see p. 34):
- train at least three times per week
- at 60–75% of maximum heart rate as outlined earlier (Karvonen principle, p. 34)
- for at least 20 minutes but ideally between 30 minutes and 2 hours, to ensure the aerobic system is working fully
- apply the principle of overload — after a few weeks your body will adapt to the exercise and resting heart rate will decrease, so to ensure you are working at 60–75% of maximum heart rate, you will have to work harder by either increasing frequency, intensity or time

- training should be specific to the requirements of the activity (it has been suggested that training should be over a distance of 2–5 times that covered in the activity)
- don't overdo it
- keep training interesting by varying the training loads, skills and activities
- your level of aerobic fitness will drop if you stop training

Fartlek training

This is a slightly different method of continuous training. The word 'fartlek' means speed-play. The pace of the run is varied to stress both the aerobic and the anaerobic energy systems. Fartlek is much more demanding and will improve an individual's VO_2(max) and recovery. A typical session lasts for 40 minutes, the intensity ranging from low to high.

Interval (intermittent) training

Interval training can be used to improve both aerobic and anaerobic capacities. It involves periods of work interspersed with recovery periods. Four main variables are used to ensure the training is specific:

- the duration of the work interval
- the intensity or speed of the work interval
- the duration of the recovery period
- the number of work intervals and recovery periods

Interval training can be adapted to overload each of the three energy systems. Anaerobic intervals should be short distance, high intensity; aerobic intervals should be long distance, submaximal intensity.

Energy system	Duration/ distance of work interval	Intensity of work interval	Duration of recovery	Number of work intervals/ recovery periods
ATP–PC	10 s/60 m	High	30 s	10
Lactic acid	35 s/200 m	High	110 s	8
Aerobic	6 min/1500 m	Submaximal	5 min	3

Strength training

Improvements in strength result from working against a resistance. The training programme should be specific to the needs of the activity. The following factors must be considered:

- the type of strength to be developed — maximum, power (elastic) or muscular endurance
- the muscle groups to be improved
- the type of muscle contraction performed in the activity — concentric, eccentric or isometric

Strength training can also be used to increase muscle growth. In this case, any exercises performed must overload the anaerobic energy systems, which will result in hypertrophy of fast-twitch fibres.

Strength can be improved by doing the following types of training:
- weights — high weights for maximum and elastic strength, low weights for muscular endurance
- circuits for muscular endurance
- plyometrics and pulleys for elastic strength

Weights
Weight training exercises are usually described in terms of sets and repetitions. The number of sets and repetitions and the amount of weight lifted depend on the type of strength to be improved.

Before designing a programme, the maximum amount of weight that the performer can lift with one repetition must be found. Then, if maximum strength is the goal, high weights with low repetitions should be lifted, e.g. 2–6 reps at 80–100% maximum strength. If muscular endurance is the goal, more repetitions of lighter weights should be done, e.g. three sets of 10 reps at 50% maximum strength.

The exercises fall into four groups:
- shoulders and arms, e.g. bench press, curls, pull-downs
- trunk and back, e.g. sit-ups, back hyperextensions
- legs, e.g. squats, calf raises, leg press
- whole body exercises, e.g. power clean, snatch, dead lift

The choice of exercise should relate to the muscle groups used in sport — both the agonists and antagonists.

Circuit training
In circuit training the athlete performs a series of exercises in succession. The exercises should include arm exercises (e.g. press-ups and triceps dips), leg exercises (e.g. squat thrusts), and trunk exercises (e.g. sit-ups and dorsal raises), as well as cardiovascular exercises such as jogging and skipping.

The athlete's body weight is used as resistance, and each exercise concentrates on a different muscle group. Circuits are usually designed for general body conditioning and are easily adapted to meet the needs of a particular activity.

Plyometrics
If leg strength is crucial to successful performance, for example in the long jump and 100 m sprint in athletics, or rebounding in basketball, then plyometrics is a method of strength training that can be used to improve power or elastic strength. It works on the concept that muscles can generate more force if they have previously been stretched. In plyometrics, on landing, the muscle performs an eccentric contraction (lengthens under tension) followed immediately by a concentric contraction as the performer jumps up. This stimulates adaptations in the neuromuscular system and results in a more powerful concentric contraction of the muscle group being worked.

Mobility (flexibility) training
Mobility training involves stretching the muscles and connective tissue. A stretch should be held for at least 10 seconds and a session should last for 10 minutes. With

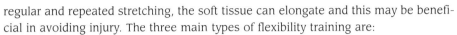

regular and repeated stretching, the soft tissue can elongate and this may be beneficial in avoiding injury. The three main types of flexibility training are:
- static stretching
- ballistic stretching
- PNF

Static stretching can be active or passive. In active stretching, the performer works on one joint, pushing it beyond its point of resistance, lengthening the muscles and connective tissue surrounding it. In passive stretching, the stretch occurs with the help of an external force, such as a partner, gravity or a wall.

Ballistic stretching involves performing a stretch with swinging or bouncing movements to push a body part even further. Only individuals who are extremely flexible, such as gymnasts and dancers, should perform this type of stretching.

PNF (proprioceptive neuromuscular facilitation) is where the muscle is contracted isometrically for a period of at least 10 seconds. It then relaxes and is stretched again, usually going further the second time.

What the examiner will expect you to be able to do
- Apply your knowledge of the training principles to practical situations.
- Calculate working intensities in terms of heart rate and Borg scale.
- Understand the importance of a warm-up and identify the different stretching exercises.
- Identify the various methods of training.
- Understand the difference between validity and reliability and apply these concepts to the various fitness tests.

Skill acquisition

Characteristics of skill

Skilled performances are:
- **learned** — the performer has spent time practising the movement
- **efficient and economical** — the movement is performed quickly and easily, without wasting energy
- **goal-directed** — the performer has a predetermined result in mind
- **fluent** — the action is smooth and movements flow together
- **aesthetic** — the action is pleasing to watch
- **consistent** — the performer is able to repeat the action successfully time after time
- **technical** — the movement matches the demonstration shown

Types of skill

The types of skill that are important in PE are:

- **motor** skills — involving movement and muscular control (e.g. performing a cartwheel)
- **cognitive** skills — involving thinking and thought processing (e.g. in badminton, a player thinks tactically and plays a long overhead clear to drive the opponent to the back of the court, followed by a drop shot)
- **perceptual** skills — involving the detection and interpretation of information (e.g. a goalkeeper in netball judges the flight of a lob pass coming into the circle and intercepts it)
- **psychomotor** skills — involving the processing of information quickly and putting decisions into action (e.g. in football, a defender sees an attacker about to make a run into space and decides to track back to block any passes to him/her)

Skill and ability

Abilities differ from skills. You need to know the differences between the two terms. Abilities are:

- **innate** — ability is genetically determined, whereas skill is learned
- **stable** and long-lasting, whereas skill can be developed and changes over time
- **foundations of skills** — you need ability to perform the skill

Performers need natural ability to reach the highest levels in sport. For example, top-level gymnasts are born with the ability of flexibility.

Types of abilities

There are two types of ability:

- **Gross motor abilities** involve movements of the large muscle groups. They relate to physical fitness and include speed, strength, stamina and suppleness/flexibility.
- **Perceptual** or **psychomotor abilities** involve sensing and interpreting information — the ability to make a judgement and put it into action.

Classification of skills

A continuum is an imaginary sliding scale on which skills can be placed between two extremes to show a gradual increase or decrease in characteristic. Continua can be used to classify skills and to develop knowledge and understanding of the characteristics of skills. This is useful in structuring practices when taking on the role of leader or coach. Classification can help us to teach, practise and improve skills in the most efficient way.

Environmental influence

Skills are classified as **open** or **closed** depending on whether the surroundings change so that the performer has to use perception to make a judgement.

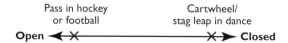

Pass in hockey or football   Cartwheel/ stag leap in dance

Open ◄─X───────────X─► Closed

You should be aware of links to the pacing continuum.

Open skills are affected by the surrounding environment, which is constantly changing. The performer must adapt to these changes — for example, movements of team-mates and the opposition. The performer must use perception and make decisions. The skill is often externally paced.

Closed skills are not affected by the environment. They can be practised in a stable environment and therefore become habitual. The skill is usually self-paced and the performer rarely uses perception.

Continuity

The **continuity** continuum classifies skills as discrete, serial or continuous.

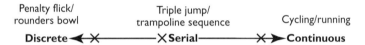

Discrete skills have a distinct beginning and ending. The performer has to start the skill from the beginning to repeat it.

Serial skills are made up of a number of discrete elements, which are combined in a particular order to form a more continuous task. Each part can be practised separately.

Continuous skills have no distinct beginning or end. The skill is often cyclic. The end of one part of the movement becomes the beginning of the next.

Muscular involvement

Skills are classified as **gross** or **fine**, depending on the number of muscles involved and the level of intricate, precise movement required.

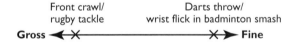

Gross skills involve movement of large muscle groups. Fine skills involve precise, intricate movements and accuracy using small muscle groups.

Pacing

The **pacing** continuum is based on who has control of the speed and timing of the skill during performance.

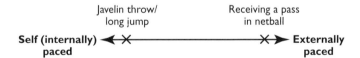

You should be aware of links to the environmental influence continuum.

If a movement is **self-paced**, the performer controls the timing, speed and rate of execution of the (usually closed) skill.

If a movement is **externally paced**, the timing, speed and rate of the skill are determined by the environment.

> **Tip** Give clear examples at the extremes of the continua — giving an example in the middle may be too vague.

Example

A tennis serve is:

- closed, because the environment remains the same
- discrete, because it has a clear beginning and ending
- gross, because it is an explosive movement and several of the major muscle groups are used
- self-paced, because the speed and timing are controlled by the performer

> **What the examiner will expect you to be able to do**
> - State the characteristics of skill and abilities — make sure you can give at least three for each. Remember that smooth and fluent for skill counts as the same point, as does innate and genetic for ability.
> - Distinguish between skill and ability — this is a common question.
> - Define the various types of skills and abilities and give examples.
> - Classify skills and justify this from your practical activities — explain how you reached your decision on where to place the skill on the continua.

Information processing

Models of information processing

You need to understand both the Whiting and the Welford models of information processing. The models use slightly different terminology but the key processes are the same.

- The **display** and **input data** from the display. The display is the sporting environment and all the information contained in it. For example, the display for a rugby player includes the ball, team-mates, opponents, pitch markings, posts, the referee and linesmen, the crowd and the coach. Some of this information will be relevant to the performer and some will be irrelevant.
- **Sense organs** or **receptor systems**. Three senses are used to detect information from the display — vision (e.g. seeing the ball and opponents), audition (e.g. hearing the shouts from the coach concerning tactics, or the crowd calling 'man on'), and proprioception, which tells us about the position of our bodies and what our muscles and joints are doing. Proprioception consists of **touch, kinaesthesis** and **equilibrium**. Kinaesthesis is the inner sense that tells us whether the movement is correct or not. Equilibrium gives information about whether the body is balanced.

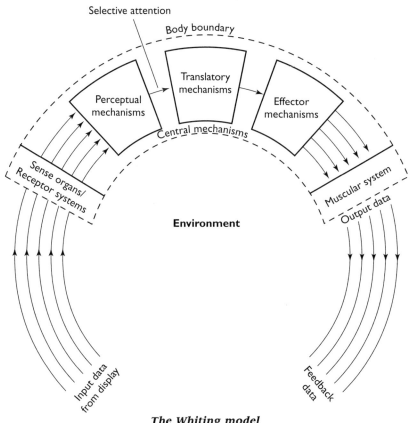

The Whiting model

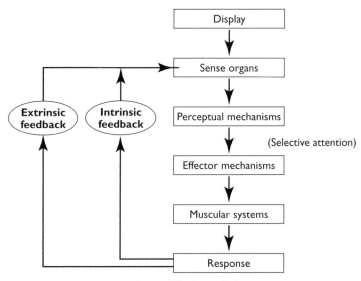

The Welford model

- **Perceptual mechanism**. This interprets the information received by the sense organs and makes a decision on what action should be taken, sometimes with the help of previous experiences stored in the memory. First, the relevant information — such as the ball, opponents and team-mates — is filtered from the irrelevant information — the crowd, linesmen etc. — by **selective attention**. Only the relevant information is acted upon; the irrelevant information is disregarded. For example, the rugby player sees a high ball and judges its speed travelling towards him. He compares it with stored memories and recognises that he has received a high ball before. Using selective attention, he focuses on the ball and disregards the crowd. He then decides on a plan of action or an appropriate response — he decides to turn sideways and jump to receive the high ball.
- **Translatory mechanism**. Using the information from the perceptual mechanism, the correct response is selected in the form of a motor programme (Whiting model only).
- **Effector mechanism**. Once the plan of action is selected, the motor programme is put into action by sending impulses through the nervous system to the relevant working muscles, enabling them to carry out the movement.
- **Muscular system**. The muscles that are needed to jump and to catch the ball receive the impulses and are ready.
- **Response** or **output data**. The movement is performed.
- **Feedback** or **feedback data**. Once the motor programme has been put into action, information about the movement is received. This could be **intrinsic** feedback (from within the performer — e.g. knowing that the ball was caught correctly because it 'feels' right, the ball is in my hands and I have landed on two feet so I feel balanced) or **extrinsic** feedback from an outside source — for example, the coach shouts 'good jump, great catch' or the crowd cheers. This information can be used to assist future performances.

The memory system

The memory system is an integral part of information processing. It stores and retrieves information, makes comparisons with previous movement experiences and selects which motor programme to retrieve in order to produce the movement.

Three components make up the **multi-store model** and you need to understand the features of each.

Short-term sensory store

The features of the short-term sensory store (STSS) are as follows:

- *All* the information (relevant and irrelevant) is held briefly — for approximately 0.25–1 second.
- It has an unlimited capacity.
- The perceptual mechanism determines which information is relevant.
- Selective attention is operational. The relevant stimuli are attended to while the irrelevant stimuli are ignored. For example, a tennis player focuses on the ball when serving and disregards the crowd. This is important because it:

- aids concentration
- improves reaction time
- filters out distractions
- controls arousal levels
- reduces the chance of information overload in the STM

Information from the STSS goes into the short-term memory.

Short-term memory

The short-term memory (STM) is the **working memory**. Its features are:
- limited storage space of 7 ± 2 items
- its capacity can be increased by '**chunking**' (see below)
- information is stored for up to 30 seconds but this can be increased with practice
- it is responsible for executing the motor programme
- information is encoded and passed to the long-term memory

> **Tip** Do not confuse the STSS and the STM.

Long-term memory (LTM)

The features of the long-term memory are as follows:
- information enters the LTM through practice
- information can be stored permanently
- it has unlimited capacity
- information is stored as motor programmes

Strategies to improve retention and retrieval

A number of strategies can be applied to help store and remember information.
- **Practice** or **rehearsal** — repetition of a skill stores the motor programme in the LTM.
- **Linking/association/past experiences** — relating new information to that already stored. For example, when learning to serve in tennis, the performer might link it to the basic over-arm throw that he/she has experienced earlier (see positive transfer on p. 57).
- **Chunking** — small pieces of information can be memorised together to extend the capacity of the STM. For example, instead of teaching a trampoline sequence as individual movements, the coach could 'chunk' three or four movements together. However, coaches should avoid giving too much information at one time because the STM can easily become overloaded.
- **Enjoyable/interesting/novel experiences** — if information is presented in a new or distinctive way, it is more likely to be remembered.
- Make it **meaningful** — if the learner understands the relevance of the skill to the performance, he/she is more likely to remember it.
- **Chaining** — information should be presented in an organised manner. For example, the elements of a tumble sequence in gymnastics should be presented in order to make it easier for the learner to remember.

- **Mental rehearsal/imagery** — visualising the skill or going over it in the mind will help the learner to remember what is needed to perform the skill. This is why demonstrations are important.
- **Reinforcement/rewards** — information is more likely to be remembered if the learner receives positive feedback or reinforcement, or is rewarded with praise after a correct response.

Reaction time

Definitions
Reaction time is the time from the onset of the stimulus to the onset of the response.

Simple reaction time is when there is one stimulus and one response. Reaction time will be very short. For example, in a swimming race the stimulus is the starter signal and the only response is to dive in.

Choice reaction time is when there are several stimuli and/or several possible responses. Reaction time will be slower. For example, in football several team-mates may be calling for a pass, and there may be several possible responses in terms of who to pass to and what type of pass.

Movement time is the time from the onset of the movement to the completion of the task.

Response time is the time from the onset of the stimulus to the completion of the task (reaction time plus movement time).

Factors affecting reaction time
A number of factors affect reaction time. They include:
- **age** — reaction time increases (slows) with age
- **gender** — generally males have faster reaction times than females
- **stimulus intensity** — if the stimulus is bright (e.g. use of pink balls in cricket) or loud (e.g. a shout), it is easier to detect and reaction time will decrease
- **temperature** — the colder the body, the slower the reaction
- **previous experience** — experience of a skill speeds up reactions
- **anticipation** — predicting a movement correctly can reduce reaction time
- **drugs and alcohol** — drugs can speed reaction time up but alcohol slows it down
- **choices** — the more choices we are presented with, the slower we react (see Hick's law)

Hick's law
Hick's law describes the impact of choice reaction time on performance. It states that while more choices make performance slower, the rate of increase in reaction time decreases with increasing choice. Hick's law is illustrated in the graph overleaf.

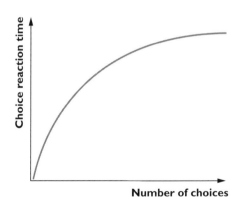

Strategies to improve the response time of a performer

There are a number of ways in which teachers and coaches can try to improve the response time of a performer. These include:

- practising responses to a stimulus (e.g. sprint starts to a gun)
- using mental rehearsal to help the performer focus on relevant information (selective attention)
- improving fitness levels
- warming up — making sure that the body and mind are prepared
- ensuring optimum arousal
- developing predictive skills — analysing the opponent's play in order to anticipate what he/she intends to do next

Psychological refractory period

Anticipation involves predicting that a movement will happen. It can be:

- **temporal**, i.e. predicting *when* the action will be performed
- **spatial**, i.e. predicting *what* action will be performed

If we anticipate correctly, then our response time will be quicker. However, if we anticipate incorrectly, our response time can be greatly increased. The diagram below illustrates what happens if we anticipate incorrectly.

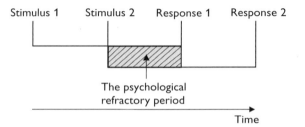

According to the **single channel hypothesis**, although we can pick up many stimuli at once, we can only *process* one piece of information at a time. Any further stimuli must wait. If we are in the middle of processing one stimulus when a second stimulus arrives, it must wait until we have finished processing the first before it can be dealt with. This delay in processing causes our reaction time to increase and is known as the **psychological refractory period**.

We can use this in sport to try to slow down the opposition. For example, in rugby you are approaching your opponent with the ball in your hands. You feign a pass to the left. This is the first stimulus and the opponent begins to move in that direction. However, you decide to play a dummy and carry on running without releasing the pass. This is the second stimulus. According to the single channel hypothesis, the opponent has to process the first stimulus of the left pass before attending to the second stimulus.

Motor programmes

A motor programme (or **executive motor programme, EMP**) is a set of movements stored in the long-term memory that specify the components of a skill. It comprises **subroutines**, which are the parts or mini skills that make up the whole skill.

Motor programmes are formed by practice. When the skill becomes grooved or over-learned, the subroutines flow together and appear to be performed automatically. This occurs when the performer reaches the **autonomous** phase of learning. Each time the motor programme is performed, it is modified and the adjustments are stored in the long-term memory.

The whole EMP is more important than the subroutines. The subroutines are **sequential** — that is, they are run in a specific order. The following diagram shows an example of a motor programme.

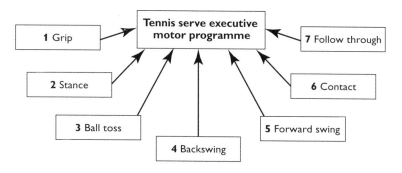

What the examiner will expect you to be able to do
- Explain sections of the Welford and/or Whiting model with the aid of practical examples.
- Draw the models and explain each component, using the same practical example throughout.
- Describe the characteristics of each of the stores in the multi-store model of memory. Remember to be specific — for example, instead of saying the STSS stores information for a small amount of time, state that it is 0.25–1 second.

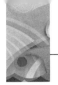

- Identify ways to improve the retrieval and storage of information *and* describe them — for example, just stating 'chunking' may not be enough to gain the mark.
- Describe the importance of selective attention to the STM — that it filters the relevant information from the irrelevant and without it the STM would overload, as it has a limited capacity of 7 ± 2 items.
- Define reaction time, movement time and response time using practical examples — use the sprint start because it is the easiest.
- Draw and label a graph of Hick's law. This is usually worth 3 marks. To gain these marks you need to show an increase on the axes, label the axes and draw the curve correctly. An increase on the axes can be shown by using numbers (e.g. 1–9) or by putting arrows on the ends of the axes.
- Describe the psychological refractory period with a practical example. Use the same example throughout — a dummy is easiest.
- Identify and describe the factors affecting reaction time. Just stating 'age' may not be enough to gain the mark — say that the older you are, the slower you will react.
- Identify a motor programme and its relevant subroutines. These should be given in sequential order to ensure you gain credit.

Learning and performance

Stages of learning

The psychologists Fitts and Posner proposed the idea of three learning phases or stages, which relate directly to the acquisition of motor skills.

The cognitive phase
This is the first stage of learning. The key points are as follows:
- The learner begins to create a mental image of what the skill should look like.
- A demonstration may be necessary.
- Mental rehearsal of the skill is required.
- The performer has to think about the skill and work out the main components.
- Trial and error is used to find the correct movement. Many mistakes are made.
- Movements might appear uncoordinated and jerky.
- The performer relies on extrinsic feedback from the coach to direct performance and highlight weaknesses. Feedback should be positive, so that the performer will persevere with the learning process.

For example, a hockey player who is learning to dribble is very slow to start with. Her movements are jerky and she often loses the ball because she hits it too hard. Her head is down and she watches the ball intently. She doesn't yet know how it is supposed to feel, so she relies on the coach for feedback. The coach gives demonstrations and the learner watches and works out each subroutine. She mentally rehearses dribbling constantly in this phase.

The associative phase

This is the intermediate stage of learning — the longest phase.

- The performer must practise.
- Demonstrations, positive feedback and mental rehearsal are still required to aid learning.
- The performer becomes more proficient and makes fewer mistakes.
- Movements become smoother and more coordinated.
- The performer begins to focus attention on the finer aspects of the skill.
- Kinaesthesis begins to develop and intrinsic feedback can be used to correct movement.
- Knowledge of results and knowledge of performance are required.
- Motor programmes develop and are stored in the long-term memory.

For example, a gymnast on a beam practises and masters the basic skills, and is able to execute more complex movements. She can now use intrinsic feedback, and is becoming aware of how the movement should feel. She can look up and forward, rather than down at her feet.

The autonomous phase

This is the final stage of learning — the expert stage.

- Movements are fluent, efficient and habitual following extensive practice.
- Skills are executed automatically without thinking about the subroutines.
- The performer can concentrate on the fine detail, tactics and advanced strategies.
- He/she uses intrinsic feedback to correct mistakes by means of kinaesthesis.
- Extrinsic feedback can be negative to aid error correction.
- Practice and mental rehearsal are important to stay at this level.

For example, a basketball player is able to dribble the ball fluently and consistently without having to look down at the ball. She is able to scan the court for passing options since the ball is controlled automatically. Errors are corrected immediately, without assistance from the coach.

Tip Questions about phases of learning are often at the beginning of the exam paper and worth 3–4 marks.

Learning curves

A learning curve illustrates the stages a performer goes though when learning a new closed skill.

- Stage 1 — the performer is in the cognitive phase of learning, so the success rate is low. The performer is trying to work out the parts of the skill and is developing an understanding.

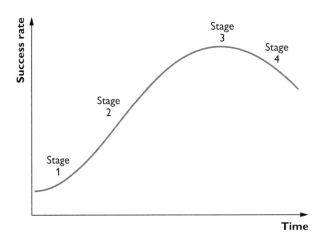

- Stage 2 — there is a sharp increase in success rate as the performer begins to grasp the skill. He/she enters the associative phase of learning and the skill begins to look more fluent. The performer's motivation levels are high as he/she is successful.
- Stage 3 — a plateau is reached where there is no improvement. The table below shows some causes of the learning plateau and solutions.

Cause	Solution
Loss of motivation/boredom	Set new tasks/challenges
	Use variable practice
	Offer tangible rewards
Mental/physical fatigue	Allow the performer to rest
	Use distributed practice
Performer has reached ability limit	Allow performer to compete against others of similar ability
Poor coaching	Try a variety of coaching methods
	Try an alternative coach
Incorrect goals set	Set goals using the SMARTER principle (see p. 58)

- Stage 4 — there is a dip in success rate. The performer lacks motivation and may experience drive reduction. A new task or challenge is required to remotivate the performer.

Motivation

Motivation is the desire to succeed. It is an individual's **drive** that inspires him/her to perform in sport.

Extrinsic motivation

Extrinsic motivation is motivation from an external source. It could be **tangible**, such as a trophy or medal, or **intangible**, such as praise from the coach.

Extrinsic reward is a valuable motivator for a beginner, but will eventually undermine intrinsic motivation. Withdrawing extrinsic rewards can lead to withdrawal from participation, especially with young performers.

Intrinsic motivation

Intrinsic motivation comes from within the performer. It is the inner drive and self-satisfaction that comes from performing.

Intrinsic motivation is longer lasting than extrinsic motivation. However, it is difficult for some performers to generate enough intrinsic motivation to continue participating in an activity.

Intrinsic motivation is less relevant at elite levels of performance.

Motivational strategies

A range of strategies can be used to maintain drive.

For cognitive performers:

- tangible, extrinsic rewards (e.g. certificates, medals, player of the match awards) will attract performers initially, and should be given periodically
- intangible extrinsic rewards (e.g. praise and positive reinforcement) will lead to increased confidence
- the activity should be fun and enjoyable
- tasks should be easily achievable to ensure success
- positive role models or significant others can help to motivate
- the health and fitness benefits of participation should be highlighted
- variable practice should be used
- collective responsibility — individuals should not be blamed for poor performances

For more advanced performers in the associative and autonomous stages:

- give praise and positive reinforcement
- generate intrinsic motivation through performance goals, for example beating a personal best
- set new, challenging goals, just within the performer's reach
- perform with an audience present
- punish lack of motivation
- use peer-group pressure

What the examiner will expect you to be able to do

- Describe the characteristics of the three phases of learning. Students often have difficulty describing the associative phase. Make sure that the practical examples you give are clear — you must be able to describe the performer's movements in each phase.
- Relate the phases of learning to feedback, guidance methods and practice methods with practical examples.

- Draw a learning curve and describe the four stages. Identify the causes of, and solutions for, the plateau.
- Define motivation and distinguish between intrinsic and extrinsic motivation, with practical examples.

Theories of learning

Operant conditioning

Connectionist or associationist theories state that learning occurs as a result of creating strong learning bonds. A learning bond is a link that connects the stimulus with the response (the **S–R bond**). The S–R bond is strengthened by **reinforcement**.

Operant conditioning is a major connectionist theory put forward by the psychologist B. F. Skinner. It suggests that an S–R bond can be created by manipulating the performer's response. A coach can accelerate the trial-and-error learning process by using strategies to:

- make the adoption of the correct response stronger
- make the neglect of the incorrect response stronger

Strategies to strengthen the S–R bond and promote adoption of the correct response include:

- allowing early success — by setting easy targets (this could include adapting the sporting environment)
- reinforcing the correct action by offering praise — if an action is not reinforced, it will not be repeated

Reinforcement

Positive reinforcement involves endorsing the performer's action when it is correct, so that the action is repeated in the future. For example, when a footballer defends a corner well, the coach offers praise in the hope that the action will be repeated in similar situations in the future.

Negative reinforcement involves the coach saying nothing when a correct action is shown, following a period of criticism about an incorrect performance. For example, a netball coach has been criticising the GA for missing shots. When the GA scores a goal, the coach says nothing. The GA recognises that she has not been criticised and repeats the correct shooting action.

Tip Do not confuse negative reinforcement with negative feedback.

Punishment is a method of reducing or eliminating undesirable actions. It can involve extra training, substitution, fines or a ban. For example, a player who drops the ball in rugby training is instructed to perform sit-ups, or a player is banned for a set period of time for constantly fouling the opposition.

Thorndike's laws

The psychologist Edward Thorndike proposed three laws to create and strengthen the S–R learning bond through the application of reinforcement.

- **Law of exercise** — the performer must practise in order to strengthen the S–R bond. If an action is not practised, the bond will weaken.
- **Law of effect** — when a correct action is shown, a satisfier such as praise should be given to strengthen the S–R bond. When an incorrect action is shown an annoyer such as criticism should be given to weaken the S–R bond.
- **Law of readiness** — an S–R bond can only be created if the performer is mentally mature enough and physically able to cope with the demands of the task.

Cognitive theories

Cognitive theories suggest that learning occurs by thinking about the task and developing a full understanding or **insight**.

Gestalt theory is the major cognitive theory. The key points are:

- skills should be taught in their entirety rather than being broken down into sub-routines — by using whole learning, the performer gains a greater understanding of the skill and develops kinaesthesis of the whole skill
- performers should think about what is required and consider the **intervening variables** (i.e. problems that can hinder performance)
- performers should use memory or insight of similar situations to help grasp the task, and use previous experience to help with the current task
- performers should use perception to make a judgement and interpret the information available

Tip Do not confuse the cognitive theory of learning and the cognitive phase of learning.

Social learning theory

The psychologist Bandura believed that we learn most effectively by copying the actions of others. The theory of **observational learning** involves watching a demonstration and replicating the model. Bandura suggested that four elements are important:

Factor	Learner	Coach
Attention	Must focus attention on the model	Can highlight the key areas of the skill
Retention	Must remember the image	Should give a clear, correct image so that it can be remembered
Motor reproduction	Must have the necessary ability and skill to replicate the demonstration	Should make sure the performer is physically capable of performing the skill
Motivation	Must have the determination to learn	Can reward or praise the performer to create the drive to learn

Learners are more likely to copy:

- **significant others** — those they respect and admire, including family members, coaches, teachers, peers and role models in the media
- models with similar characteristics (e.g. age, gender)
- actions that are successful
- actions that are reinforced

Schmidt's schema theory

Schema theory suggests that the same skills can be used in different sports because the performer develops a set of 'generalised movements' that allow skills to be adapted to suit the situation. This is why some performers are capable in many sports. The schema has two parts:

- the **recall schema** stores information and initiates the movement
- the **recognition schema** controls and evaluates the movement

The performer's experience draws together information from four areas, or **memory items**:

- The initial conditions — the player gathers information from the environment, such as the position of other players. For example, a centre player in netball has the ball in her hands and is on the edge of the shooting circle. The GS is unmarked to her left. She remembers being in a similar situation both in training and in previous games.
- The response specification is based on the initial conditions. The player decides what movement to do. She decides to send a short, flat, fast pass to the GS, as she is quite near, before her defender recovers her position.
- The sensory consequences — the player gathers sensory information about the movement using intrinsic feedback or kinaesthesis. As she passes the ball, she feels her elbows bend and knows that as the ball left her hands it felt correct. She placed enough power and height on the pass.
- The response outcomes gather information about the result of the movement. Was it successful or unsuccessful? For example, the GS received the pass and went on to score a goal.

Developing schemas

Coaches can organise practices to enable schemata to develop by:

- ensuring that practice is **varied** — to build a range of experience
- ensuring that practised skills are **transferable** from training to the game situation
- giving **feedback** to help improve skills
- giving **praise** and positive reinforcement
- **practising** a range of skills until they are well-learned

Transfer of learning

Transfer explains the effect that the learning of one skill may have on the learning of another skill. Nearly all learning is based on some form of transfer.

- **Positive transfer** occurs when the learning of one skill facilitates the learning of another skill — for example, two skills that have a similar form: learning to throw in a rugby union line-out helps with long passing in American football.
- **Negative transfer** occurs when the learning of one skill inhibits the learning of an additional skill — for example, a netball player may not dribble when playing basketball because she transfers the static footwork rule across the two sports.
- **Proactive transfer** occurs when a previously learned skill has an effect on a skill learned later. It can be positive or negative. For example, learning to serve in volleyball now will (positively) affect the learning of a tennis serve in the future.
- **Retroactive transfer** occurs when new skills influence the learning and performance of a skill learned previously. This can also be positive or negative. For example, learning a golf drive may affect a hockey stroke (negatively) when you go back to playing hockey, because your swing is too high.
- **Bilateral transfer** is the transfer of skills from one side of the body to the opposite side. For example, learning how to perform snooker shots with one hand and then transferring to the other hand.
- **Zero transfer** occurs when there are no similarities between the tasks and therefore no effect on either skill. For example, learning to Eskimo roll in a canoe and learning an overhead clear in badminton will have no effect on each other.

To ensure positive transfer the coach should:
- ensure that the performer's first skill is grooved
- highlight the potential for transfer
- ensure that the practice environment for both skills is similar
- make practice sessions as close to the game situation as possible
- give praise, reinforcement and rewards when positive transfer takes place

To limit the effects of negative transfer the coach should:
- ensure that the first skill is grooved before the second skill is presented
- highlight the differences in the skills, and therefore the potential for negative transfer
- ensure that the performer understands all the components of the skill

You should be aware of the link between schema theory and transfer of learning. When a performer transfers learning from one skill to another, he/she builds a range of experiences and is able to adapt his/her motor programmes and performance to suit other environmental situations. An adapted motor programme is called a schema. Some performers appear to have a natural sporting ability, enabling them to be proficient in a number of skills and sports. They are *transferring* skills and using their experiences of other sports to help in the current situation.

Goal setting

Research has shown that setting goals has a positive effect on performance. The benefits of setting goals include:
- giving the performer an aim or focus
- increasing motivation

- increasing confidence levels
- controlling arousal levels
- focusing efforts in training and game situations

Types of goal

There are three types of goal:
- **process goals** are set to improve technique
- **performance goals** are set to improve personal bests
- **product** or **outcome goals** are based on winning

Principles of goal setting

When setting goals the SMARTER principle should be applied:
- **S**pecific — goals should be specific and detailed, for example reaching level 10.5 on the multi-stage fitness test.
- **M**easurable — goals must be quantifiable, for example making ten tackles in the next half.
- **A**greed — goals must be concurred by the performer and the coach so that they have shared responsibility for achieving the goal, for example you and your coach deciding to reduce your 400 m time by 2 seconds.
- **R**ealistic — goals have to be within the performer's reach, for example aiming to run your first 10 km in under 55 minutes.
- **T**ime phased — a set period must be stated in which the goal should be reached, for example performing a personal best time in the 100 m freestyle by the end of next month.
- **E**xciting — the goal has to be motivational, for example learning to do a somersault on the trampoline by next week.
- **R**ecorded — the progress has to be written down, for example the coach should document the height of every high jump you make so that progress can be evaluated.

What the examiner will expect you to be able to do
- Describe the three theories of learning and explain how a performer learns a skill using each method.
- State Thorndike's laws and explain how they strengthen the S–R bond.
- Describe and give examples of positive and negative reinforcement.
- Critically evaluate the theories of learning, supporting your answers with practical examples.
- Identify the four memory items of a schema and explain them using a practical example (use the same example throughout).
- Understand the link with varied and realistic practices in the development of schemata.
- Describe and give examples of the various types of transfer — make sure you give clear examples, particularly with proactive and retroactive transfer.
- Show knowledge of the importance of transfer in developing schemata.

- Explain the benefits of setting goals and the SMARTER principle — don't forget the practical examples.
- Discuss the types of goals — stick to one example throughout product, performance and process goals, to illustrate your knowledge.

Skill acquisition in practical situations

Factors to consider when coaching

The style of teaching and the type of guidance offered can determine the success of a training session and greatly influence the motivation and enjoyment levels of the performer. When planning training sessions, the coach should consider:
- the experience level of the performers/what phase of learning they are in
- the fitness levels of the performers
- whether the task is dangerous
- the classification of the skills being taught in terms of environmental influence, pacing etc.
- the level of motivation of the performers
- the size of the group

Teaching styles

Command style

In the command style of teaching, the coach instructs the group and is in full control. The coach makes *all* the decisions. It is best used:
- in dangerous situations
- when time is limited
- with cognitive performers
- with large groups
- with a task that has one correct response
- when the learner is fully aware of what is required

Disadvantages of the command style are:
- it discourages creativity
- there is no differentiation in tasks for different abilities
- learners may become bored and demotivated

Reciprocal style

In the reciprocal style of teaching, the coach delegates some of the teaching to the more able members of the group. The advantages are:
- increased contact and communication between group members
- it is useful with mixed ability groups
- all ability levels develop, either as 'coach' or learner

- feedback is given instantly as there may be several 'coaches'
- coaches may develop new ideas

Disadvantages of the reciprocal style include:
- it is time-consuming
- student coaches may lack experience
- student coaches may instruct or demonstrate incorrectly

Problem solving or discovery style

The problem solving or discovery style involves the coach posing an open task for the learners to work through, discovering how to solve the problem in their own way in their own time. Advantages include:
- increased contact and communication between group members
- it is useful with mixed ability groups
- it is motivational, since learners achieve at their own level
- creativity is encouraged

Disadvantages of the problem solving or discovery style are:
- it is time-consuming
- incorrect techniques can be developed
- it is difficult to give feedback to large groups
- there are safety implications of allowing learners to work independently

Methods of presenting practice

To decide on the best method of presenting a skill to the learner, the coach first has to consider the classification and organisation of the movement. The best practice method will allow the skill to become grooved or over-learned.

Whole practice

Whole practice involves teaching the skill in its entirety. It is the best method for skills that are highly organised and cannot easily be broken down into separate subroutines. Examples include continuous skills, such as cycling and jogging, and simple, discrete skills where a single action is required, such as a forward roll.
- Whenever possible, skills should be taught as a whole, to develop the correct feel of the skill (kinaesthesis).
- It saves time in that there is no assembling of the parts.
- The performer gains a clear mental image of the whole skill, which can easily be transferred into real game situations.
- It is the best method for ballistic actions that cannot be broken down, for example a golf swing.
- It is the best method for performers in the autonomous phase of learning.

Part practice

In part practice the skill is broken down into its subroutines and each part is practised until it is flawless. This method is best for skills that are low in organisation and easily broken down into subroutines. It is also useful for serial skills, as each of the discrete elements can be practised independently.

- It is good for cognitive learners because just part of the skill can be focused on, reducing the chance of overload.
- It can reduce fatigue in physically demanding skills. For example, the correct leg kick in front crawl could be the focus of teaching rather than the entire skill.
- It is useful when the task is complex or dangerous.
- It allows the performer to build confidence and increases motivation.
- It aids understanding of complex tasks, since the skill is broken down.

Progressive part method

Progressive part practice (sometimes called 'chaining') attempts to solve one of the problems of part practice by maintaining the links between subroutines. The first subroutine or part of the skill is taught and practised until perfect. The other parts are then added sequentially until the whole skill can be performed. Progressive part practice is useful when teaching the main components of the triple jump, for example.

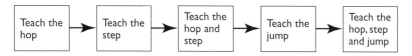

Whole–part–whole practice

This method involves performing the whole skill and identifying any weaknesses. The weaker parts are practised in isolation and then integrated back into the whole skill. It is useful for learners performing complex tasks and for more experienced performers who may be encountering problems. For example, when teaching front crawl:

- the whole skill is introduced initially
- the arm action is practised in isolation with the aid of floats
- the whole skill is practised again with improved arm action

Types of practice

Variable practice

In variable practice, the environment is constantly changing. Therefore it is best for open skills. An example is changing from partner work to unopposed practice to three-versus-two in rugby — the players can therefore develop their passing techniques and positional skills, which can be transferred directly into a game situation. Benefits of variable practice include:

- performers learn to respond to the changing environment
- decision-making and perceptual skills develop
- adaptations are stored and therefore the experience of the performer is expanded
- it improves selective attention

Massed practice

Massed practice is continuous practice without rest periods. It is a useful method for improving discrete, closed or simple skills. The continuous method helps to groove or over-learn skills so that they become habitual. It can be physically demanding, so is most effective with highly motivated or autonomous performers. A high level of fitness is essential, although it may be used to develop fitness in lower level performers. Examples include a badminton player trying to perfect a short serve, and a trampolinist continuously practising a seat drop to make it habitual.

Distributed practice

Distributed practice is practice with rest periods included. The physical practice time is often less than the rest period. This method is regarded as more effective than massed practice. It is useful for practising continuous, dangerous, complex or tiring skills. The breaks in performance allow for physical recovery, so it is useful for performers who lack physical fitness. The rest periods allow time for mental practice. Distributed practice can also be used with cognitive performers, the coach giving feedback during the rest periods. An example of distributed practice is a steeplechaser running laps of a running track followed by a rest period, during which he/she mentally rehearses the performance — seeing the stride pattern, clearing the barriers and the water barrier.

Mental practice

Mental practice involves the performer going over the task in his/her mind without moving. It has been found to improve reaction times and confidence and may increase motivation. The best improvements in performance are made when physical practice is combined with mental rehearsal.

Methods of guidance

There are four types of guidance that can be used to help the learning process.

Verbal guidance involves the coach instructing the performers in the key points of the skill — telling them what to do and how to do it.
- It is often used in conjunction with visual guidance.
- It is useful for more advanced performers in the autonomous stage of learning.
- It can be given during a performance.
- It is useful for open skills, where the performer needs to make decisions and adapt quickly.
- It can be used to give tactical, strategic or technical information that a cognitive performer may not understand.
- Information should be kept brief and meaningful to avoid overload.

Visual guidance involves the performer *seeing* the correct method of performing the skill.
- It could be a demonstration by the coach, a video, a skill card or a coaching manual.
- It is effective for performers in the cognitive stage of learning.
- It helps to build a clear mental picture of how the skill should be performed.
- The performer can grasp the key components of the movement as his/her attention is focused.
- The coach can change or modify the display — for example, placing a chalked square on a tennis court for the performer to aim for while practising serves.

Manual guidance involves the coach holding and physically 'shaping' the body to give the learner an idea of how the skill should feel. **Mechanical guidance** involves the use of a piece of equipment or a device to aid and shape movement. Both these methods:
- are effective for performers in the cognitive stage
- are useful in dangerous tasks as they improve safety
- reduce fear and anxiety and therefore build confidence
- allow the whole skill to be attempted
- allow the performer to develop kinaesthesis

The drawbacks include:
- the performer may become reliant on the support/aid
- incorrect kinaesthesis could develop
- bad habits might be instilled
- the performer might become demotivated by feeling that he/she is not performing the skill alone
- the physical contact or proximity of the coach may make the performer feel uncomfortable

Types of feedback

Feedback is the information received about the skill by the performer during the course of a movement, or as a result of it. Feedback plays a vital role in correcting errors and improving performance. There are several different types of feedback you need to be aware of. These are summarised in the tables below:

Intrinsic feedback	Extrinsic feedback
Comes from within (e.g. proprioceptors and kinaesthesis)	Comes from external sources (e.g. coach, team-mates, crowd)
Concerns the feel of the movement (e.g. the feeling of balance during a headstand)	Received via sight and hearing
Begins to develop in the associative phase of learning	Cognitive performers rely on extrinsic feedback since they haven't yet developed kinaesthesis
Autonomous performers use it to correct errors	Importance of developing intrinsic feedback should be highlighted to cognitive performers

Positive feedback	Negative feedback
Received when the movement is correct, to reinforce the action	Received when the movement is incorrect, to stop the incorrect action from being repeated
Can be intrinsic or extrinsic	Can be intrinsic or extrinsic
Used to motivate performers	Reduces the chance of bad habits developing
Essential for cognitive performers (e.g. a coach praising a novice hurdler for a quick trail leg action)	Used with more advanced performers who may begin to detect their own errors

Knowledge of performance	Knowledge of results
Concerns the quality of the performance	Concerns the outcome of the performance
Technique based — tells you *why* the movement was correct or incorrect	Results based — was the movement successful or unsuccessful?
Can be intrinsic or extrinsic	Can be positive or negative
Used by experienced performers as they use kinaesthesis	Important for cognitive performers

Concurrent	Terminal	Delayed
Continuous feedback received during the movement	Feedback received when the movement has finished	Feedback given at a later date
Can be intrinsic (kinaesthesis) or extrinsic (the coach giving instructions as you perform)	Extrinsic	Extrinsic
Autonomous	Cognitive/autonomous	Autonomous

What the examiner will expect you to be able to do
- Identify the factors to consider before leading or coaching a practical session.
- Describe the various teaching styles and suggest advantages and disadvantages for each.
- Describe the various methods of practice and relate them to classification.
- Link the methods of practice to the three phases of learning.
- Critically evaluate each of the methods of practice, giving advantages and disadvantages of each, and support your answers with practical examples.
- Critically evaluate each of the methods of guidance, giving advantages and disadvantages of each, and support your answer with practical examples.
- Explain the various types of feedback, with examples, and relate them to the phases of learning.
- Discuss the benefits and functions of feedback.

Opportunities for participation
Concepts

This section introduces some of the concepts, categorisations and benefits of physical activity to individuals and society. The key characteristics are features that help identify a particular concept. The objectives are the aims or functions of a concept for individuals or society in general.

Leisure time

Key characteristics

Leisure can be defined as spare time during which individuals can choose what to do. When all duties and obligations have been completed, there may be a little time left to spend as you wish. Some people like to relax and spend their free time inactively, while others look for excitement and danger — it is a matter of personal choice.

Key objectives

Functions of leisure for an individual can be summarised by a number of 's words':
- **s**tress relief — relaxation, improve health and fitness
- **s**ocial benefits — meeting people, forming friendships
- physical **s**kill development
- **s**elf-confidence and **s**elf-fulfilment improvement

Leisure time used in a positive way also has a number of functions for society. It:
- encourages conformity
- civilises society
- encourages social and racial mixing

Physical recreation

Key characteristics

Recreation can be defined as the **active** aspect of leisure. It is entered into voluntarily during free time and people have a choice concerning which activities to take part in. The focus is on **participation** rather than results.

Key objectives

Recreation provides many benefits for individuals, including the opportunity to:
- relax
- socialise
- be creative
- improve health and fitness

Recreation can also be said to increase conformity and morality in society as a whole. Social benefits of recreation include:
- community integration through mass participation events
- less strain on the NHS
- social control and crime reduction
- employment opportunities
- economic benefits

Play

Key characteristics

A useful way of remembering the key features of play is to use the mnemonic 'TESCO':
- **T**ime and space are flexible
- **E**njoyment
- **S**pontaneous
- **C**hild-like
- **O**ptional whether you play or not

Key functions of play

Play has many different functions both for adults and children.

The key feature of adult play is **motive**. For an adult, play has mainly psychological benefits as it can provide stress relief, an escape from the reality of everyday life, and an opportunity to relax.

The main function of play for children is to **master reality**. Through play, children can learn:

- social skills, such as making friends and cooperation
- physical skills, such as coordination
- emotional skills, such as accepting defeat
- environmental skills, such as safety awareness
- cognitive skills, such as decision-making
- moral skills, such as fair play

Comparing and contrasting play and recreation

For the Unit 1 exam, it is important that you are able to identify shared characteristics of certain concepts, as well showing knowledge of differences between them.

Characteristics shared by play and recreation include the following:

- They are entered into of one's own free will.
- The primary motivation is enjoyment.
- They have an informal structure — for example, flexible rules and time.
- The outcome is non-serious, and a casual attitude is adopted.

Differences between play and physical recreation include the following:

- While intrinsic motivation is the primary aim for both play and recreation, other motives are likely to be involved in the recreation process — adults may use recreation to escape the stresses of daily life, and view it as an opportunity to improve their health and wellbeing.
- While both play and recreation have a flexible, loose organisation or structure, recreation is slightly more organised than play.

Sport

Key characteristics

Sport is different from play and physical recreation in that it is competitive, strict rules apply and extrinsic rewards are available for winning. The more you can identify features such as competition, high skill levels and physical exertion, the more likely it is that the activity can be classified as sport.

Sport is:

- **s**erious/competitive — the aim is to win, with the 'win at all costs' attitude or sportsmanship
- **p**rowess — high skill levels, particularly by professionals and elite performers, commitment to train/improve
- **o**rganised — sport has strict rules and regulations, NGBs setting rules
- **r**ewards — available for winning (extrinsic) and intrinsic satisfaction
- **t**ime and space restrictions apply, as sport is far more structured and organised

Key functions

Sport serves a number of important functions for individuals including:

- improved health and fitness
- increased self-esteem and self-confidence
- opportunities for socialising

Comparing physical recreation and sport

Physical recreation	High-level sport
Immediate pleasure	Sometimes enjoyable, particularly in victory, but may involve anxiety and pain
Participation provides intrinsic rewards and enjoyment	There may be extrinsic rewards
Length of participation is the individual's choice	Time constraints on training and length of game
Spontaneity exists	Less spontaneous because of game plans
Level of training is the individual's choice	Serious training is required
Flexible rule	Strict rules

Outdoor and adventurous activities

Outdoor and adventurous activities (OAA) form one of the six areas of National Curriculum PE (outdoor education) but are also important as outdoor recreation.

Characteristics of OAA as outdoor education

OAA as outdoor education can be defined as 'the achievement of educational objectives via guided and direct experiences in the natural environment'. For example, pupils who are up a mountain and being formally instructed in skills such as map reading and taking a compass bearing are taking part in outdoor and adventurous activity in PE.

Functions of OAA in the National Curriculum

OAA have many functions, including raising awareness of and respect for oneself, others, the natural environment and danger or risk. Risks should be perceived only (i.e. in a pupil's head) rather than real (actual danger).

Outdoor activities such as hill walking, caving and canoeing can give personal challenges to individuals, as well as teaching them how to work effectively with one another (teamwork, cooperation). They can provide opportunities to experience the responsibilities of leadership, such as making decisions that affect the rest of the group. Communication skills and an awareness of an individual's strengths and weaknesses may develop.

A sense of adventure and excitement is an important part of the outdoor experience.

Outdoor activities need to be specifically linked to the natural environment (e.g. mountain walking and rock climbing). Such activities as part of compulsory National

Curriculum PE belong under the overall umbrella of PE, and so involve the same potential set of values (physical skills, health and fitness improvement, social and cognitive development).

Factors influencing a pupil's OAA experience

OAA in most schools tends to be of relatively low quality. A number of factors may negatively affect a pupil's OAA experience:

- If staff lack specialist qualifications, experience or motivation, the opportunities for a positive and meaningful experience will be reduced.
- Lessons do not allow much time for OAA.
- Access or transport to the natural environment is a problem for many schools.
- Money and resources — the expense of undertaking OAA may be too much for many schools and parents. Specialist equipment may not be readily available.
- Parents and teachers are likely to be deterred by the inherent risks of certain activities such as skiing and mountain climbing.

It is important to be able to give a critical evaluation of a pupil's OAA experience in relation to the factors identified above, and to appreciate that in many schools it is taught in a limited manner due to such factors. For example, orienteering activities may be restricted to the school grounds.

Key characteristics of OAA as outdoor recreation

The characteristics and functions of physical recreation are defined and explained on p. 65. The key distinguishing feature of outdoor recreation is that it takes place in the natural environment, for example climbing a mountain or canoeing down a fast-flowing river.

Key functions of OAA as outdoor recreation

Individuals who choose to participate in outdoor recreation activities do so to:

- improve health and fitness
- relieve stress and relax
- develop self-esteem and self-confidence (personal challenge)
- develop an appreciation of the natural environment
- develop cognitive skills and decision-making abilities
- develop social skills and work as a team
- develop survival skills

Increased participation in OAA as outdoor recreation

In general, people nowadays have more free time and more disposable income than in previous generations. The early twenty-first century has seen continued interest in spending this extra time and money pursuing various outdoor recreation activities. Reasons for choosing outdoor recreation as leisure time activities include:

- the positive portrayal by the media — snow boarding and mountain biking, for example, are seen as cool
- an increased desire for excitement — the adrenaline rush
- participation is non-competitive

> **What the examiner will expect you to be able to do**
> - Show understanding of the characteristics and objectives of a range of concepts — in isolation and compared to and contrasted with one another.
> - Explain the benefits of sport and leisure to individuals as well as to society in general. This is sometimes linked to government or local authority provision.

Current provision for active leisure

You need to know the characteristics and aims of the public, private and voluntary sectors in relation to active leisure provision in the UK.

Public sector provision

The important features of public sector provision (e.g. leisure centres, swimming pools, public parks) include:
- facilities are open to all, non-exclusive
- run by local authorities and managed by local authority employees
- run as business operations, with the aim of breaking even
- trade on set prices according to pre-set budgets
- facilities and services are of adequate or improving standard

Aims

Central government sees the provision of facilities for sport and recreation as increasingly important in today's society because of health and obesity issues. By providing facilities and schemes to increase participation in physical activity, local authorities aim to:
- increase health and fitness of individuals and improve the health and wellbeing of the community
- increase social control and reduce crime in the community
- improve social integration
- provide for social needs, equal opportunities and social inclusion
- regenerate areas (this may link to national government policy)

Such aims need to be achieved within financial constraints. Local authorities are required to break even and to give taxpayers value for money.

Private sector provision

Private sector leisure provision, such as the David Lloyd health clubs, have the following characteristics:
- they are exclusive, with a selective clientele — elitist
- they are privately owned or belong to registered companies
- they trade on profit-and-loss accounts — the main aim is to make a profit

- they are managed by owners or appointed employees
- they offer a high-quality service and facilities (at a price!)

Membership of private fitness clubs has become increasingly attractive to the general public in our health-conscious society.

Advantages of private fitness clubs are that individuals have more choice of where to go to improve their health and fitness, with such clubs offering high-quality facilities and service to encourage continued participation. Personal trainers may help individuals with low levels of fitness or self-motivation. However, such high-quality provision is too expensive for the majority, who rely instead on cheaper alternatives within the public and voluntary sectors. Sometimes individuals are deterred from private-sector participation because it is viewed as elitist and exclusively for the rich.

Aims
The key aims of private sector provision are to:
- make a profit
- increase membership numbers
- provide an exclusive, high-quality service for members

Voluntary sector provision

Voluntary sector sports clubs, such as local athletics, rugby and tennis clubs, are:
- run by members or committees on a voluntary basis (this reduces costs and overheads)
- sometimes owned by members on a trust or charity basis
- financed by membership fees, fund-raising etc.
- run on a profit-and-loss basis — making a profit is not an overriding concern

Aims
Key aims of voluntary sector leisure provision are to:
- provide for grass-roots sports participation
- increase club membership and performance levels
- provide opportunities for people to meet others with similar interests
- seek funds from sponsors and the lottery to develop playing opportunities and facilities

Best value

'Best value' is a key government policy requiring local authorities and other related organisations to provide the best value for money possible. It is the principle on which local authorities decide who should run a particular service — who can provide the highest quality service at the best possible price.

'Best value' is the principle in operation in the public sector aiming to increase accountability and provide a higher quality of service for users of public-sector provision. Existing local authorities and private sector companies can bid to run sport and leisure services and offer 'best value' in doing so.

> **What the examiner will expect you to be able to do**
> - Know and understand:
>   - the characteristics and goals of the public, private and voluntary sectors
>   - the advantages and disadvantages of the public, private and voluntary sectors
>   - the concept of 'best value' in relation to public sector provision for sport/ recreation
> - Identify the key characteristics of a particular sector and compare the different sectors.
> - Understand the changing relationship between the public and private sectors in relation to provision for active leisure.

Increasing participation: the role of schools and national governing bodies

Historical, social and cultural factors

Legacy of the nineteenth-century public schools

The National Curriculum for PE emphasises the importance of team games in developing qualities such as sportsmanship, teamwork and leadership in individuals. Learning how to be competitive is an important part of modern life. Respecting opponents and officials are key aims today, as they were in earlier times. Fair play and sportsmanship are seen as positive qualities that can be developed through PE at school. Improved decision-making and cognitive skills are also seen as important values resulting from involvement in team games.

Success in sport can raise the status of a school and can be used as a marketing tool to promote the school. Many schools have competitive fixtures with other schools, as well as their own house systems, and some have established traditions of excellence.

Development of PE in elementary state schools

You need to understand the following key terms:
- **Objectives:** reasons why different syllabuses were introduced and what they were trying to achieve (*aims*)
- **Content:** *what* was being taught in a lesson
- **Methodology:** *how* a lesson was taught (and at times by whom?)

The Model Course 1902

Colonel Fox of the War Office introduced the Model Course of Physical Training in 1902. It had a military emphasis with no educational focus and did not cater for children's needs. Its intention of improving the health and fitness of the children was questionable. The exercises were mainly static and dull. It lasted for just 2 years.

Objectives	Content	Methodology
• to improve fitness (for military service) • training in the handling of weapons • to improve discipline	• military drill • exercises in unison • weapon training	• command–response (e.g. 'Attention', 'Stand at ease', 'Marching, about turn') • group response, no individuality • in ranks

Early developments in physical training (1904 and 1909 syllabuses)

Dr George Newman was a key influence in the development of the PT syllabuses. He was appointed as Chief Medical Officer to the Board of Education. As a doctor, he was interested in the health-giving effects of exercise.

Objectives	Content	Methodology
• therapeutic effects of exercise, with emphasis on respiration, circulation and posture • obedience and discipline still important • enjoyment • alertness, decision-making, control of mind over body	• Swedish in character, with recreational aspects to relieve the tedium and monotony of former drill-style lessons • dancing steps and simple games	• 1904: 109 tables of exercises for teachers to follow • 1909: reduced to 71 tables • still formal, in ranks, with marching and free-standing exercises • still group response to commands • a kinder approach by teachers, some freedom of choice for teachers

1919 syllabus

Objectives	Content	Methodology
• enjoyment and play for the under-7s • therapeutic work for the over-7s • age differentiation starting to appear in PT lessons	• the exercises performed were similar to those in 1909 syllabus • a special section of games for the under-7s was included • not less than half the lesson was spent on 'general activity exercises' — active free movement, including small games and dancing	• more freedom for teachers and pupils • less formal than previous PT syllabuses

1933 syllabus

The 1933 PT syllabus was seen as a watershed between the syllabuses of the past and the physical education of the future.

Objectives	Content	Methodology
• physical fitness • therapeutic results • good physique and posture • development of mind and body (holistic development)	• athletics, gymnastics and games skills • group work	• still direct style for the majority of the lesson • some decentralised parts to the lesson • group work/tasks throughout • special PE clothing worn during lessons • many schools now had specialist facilities available (e.g. newly built gymnasiums)

Development of state PE in the 1950s

Moving and Growing was produced in 1952 by the Education Department as a guide for primary schools. Primary school teachers were not trained in physical education, so they needed guidance to plan and deliver it. The term 'physical education' had evolved, giving a different emphasis from the earlier 'physical training'.

Rudolf Laban influenced the development of state PE in the 1950s with his work on movement to music, educational dance and creativity. His work became highly influential in *Moving and Growing* (1952) and *Planning the Programme* (1954).

Objectives of PE in the 1950s	Content of PE in the 1950s	Methodology of PE in the 1950s
• to develop physical, social and cognitive skills • variety of experiences in a fun atmosphere • increased involvement for everyone, at their own level of ability	• agility exercises, gymnastics, dance and games skills • swimming • movement to music	• child-centred and enjoyment orientated • progressive • teacher guidance rather than direction • problem-solving, creative, exploratory, discovery • individual interpretation of tasks encouraged • using apparatus in lessons — ropes, bars, boxes, mats

The start of a 'recreational focus'

In the last decades of the twentieth century, radical changes were made to the physical activities in state schools. The Butler Education Act 1944 required local authorities to provide recreational sporting facilities in schools. This was a very different philosophy from the one held at the beginning of the twentieth century, which believed that the working classes had no need for recreation. The secondary school teacher was now fully trained and therefore no longer dependent on following a syllabus drawn up centrally. Physical education teachers were to experience 40 years of a decentralised system, where they had autonomy and were able to choose their own physical education programmes.

National Curriculum PE

By the end of the 1980s, the government wanted:
- more control of education
- more teacher accountability
- national standards for physical education
- a wider range of activities to be taught

The 1988 Education Reform Act led to the introduction of National Curriculum physical education, which applies to all state schools. This represented a return to a centralised approach towards education. All state schools now follow set guidelines for set subjects to teach, which are inspected by Ofsted.

PE was made compulsory for all 5–16-year-olds, reinforcing its importance. Through physical education, children should be able to:
- achieve physical competence (i.e. improve physical skills)
- improve self-confidence and knowledge of strengths and weaknesses
- perform in a range of activities, including those that encourage active leisure
- improve health and fitness
- become a 'critical performer' (i.e. children should be encouraged to observe and analyse physical activities in a knowledgeable way)
- learn how to plan, perform and evaluate
- improve cognitive skills and decision-making
- improve social skills and leadership qualities

Critical performer
The National Curriculum aims to provide students with knowledge of roles in sport other than performer. Roles such as official, coach, spectator and leader encourage students to appreciate physical activities in different ways, and possibly to take on some of these roles at various stages of their lives.

Areas of activity
The current aims of PE are to offer a broad range of physical activities. Concentrating on one activity would not provide a balanced physical development. The National Curriculum classifications are:
- games
- athletics
- swimming
- gymnastics
- dance
- outdoor and adventurous activities

Schools cannot offer every sport available but there should be a balance of activities — team and individual, competitive and non-competitive — selected from the categories listed above.

Factors that influence PE and sport provision in schools

A pupil's experience of PE and sport at school can be positive or negative, depending on various factors in individual schools.

- Timetable restrictions. Schools sometimes reduce the amount of time allocated to PE due to the demands of other, more 'academic' subjects. PE may be marginalised, particularly at Key Stage 4 when the demands of GCSE examinations are high.
- Lack of funding or resources. Budgets may restrict the quality and breadth of a pupil's PE experience. For example, many schools find the funding of swimming and OAA particularly difficult. Transport for fixtures might also be deemed too expensive and could negatively affect inter-school sporting opportunities.
- Quality of staffing. PE teachers and external coaches vary in terms of qualifications and their degree of commitment to PE/school sport.
- Quality of facilities. The availability of specialist facilities for offering a range of PE and sport varies throughout the country.
- School–club links. Links between schools and clubs can positively influence PE and school sport, by improving a pupil's access to high-quality coaching and facilities.

As well as the core curriculum lessons, children are offered many other sporting experiences at school. Extra-curricular activities are optional activities offered in schools during lunchtime and after school. They offer recreational experiences as well as competitive fixtures. This is also called school sport, which should be differentiated from physical education. Physical education refers to the compulsory core lessons.

In the UK, physical education and school sport have traditionally been kept separate, as they are believed to serve different aims. However, there is now a growing belief that these two strands should be brought closer together and initiatives are taking place to try to achieve this. Examples include the Physical Education, School Sport and Club Links (PESSCL) strategy and sports college status being given to some schools.

Current government policies

PE, School Sport and Club Links strategy

PESSCL is a national strategy aimed at increasing the uptake of sporting opportunities by 5–16-year-olds so that 85% of them experience a minimum of 2 hours' high-quality PE and school sport each week.

Sports colleges

Sports colleges are part of the specialist schools programme run by the Department for Children, Schools and Families. Sports colleges help to deliver the government's plans for PE and sport. They provide high-quality opportunities for young people in their neighbourhood.

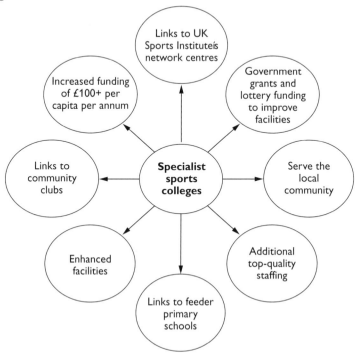

Club Links

A school–club link is an agreement between a school or school sport partnership and a community-based sports club to work together to:

- meet the needs of all young people who might want to get involved in their sport/club
- help young people to realise their ambitions in sport and dance by providing pathways for them to follow
- provide new and varied opportunities for people
- agree good standards of provision, putting in place quality controls to ensure that standards remain high

The main aim of the Club Links programme is to increase the number of children participating in sports clubs.

National governing bodies: increasing participation

National governing bodies (NGBs) are required to open their sport to all sections of society, including those at grass-roots participation levels. Ways of achieving increased participation include:

- developing policies linking to specific target groups (e.g. people with disabilities, ethnic minorities)
- training more sport-specific coaches to encourage participation

- developing mini-games and modified versions of their sports to encourage partic-ipation at all levels of ability (e.g. high 5 netball, short tennis)
- making facilities more accessible, affordable and attractive and targeting funds at grass-roots levels and inner-city schemes
- improving awareness of the sport through publicity, advertising and use of positive role models

Sport England

Sport England is a government-funded agency responsible for developing a world-class community sports system. It published a new strategy in June 2008, designed to get more people playing and enjoying sport.

Its key aims are to:
- encourage a million more individuals to do more sport (e.g. via free swimming)
- decrease by 25% the number of 16-year-olds dropping out of sports
- improve talent development in at least 25 sports
- support the 'Five-Hour Sport' offer for children and young people (e.g. through the Sports Unlimited initiative and school–club links)

Sport England has three clear outcomes:
- **grow** — increasing participation
- **sustain** — maintaining participation
- **excel** — developing talent support systems

Sports Leaders UK

Sports Leaders UK provides the opportunity and motivation for people to make a meaningful contribution to their local community through nationally recognised sports leadership awards. Two examples are:
- The Junior Sports Leadership Award for 14–16-year-olds, taught mainly within the National Curriculum for PE at Key Stage 4. The award develops young people's skills in organising activities, planning, communicating and motivating.
- The Community Sports Leadership Award, designed for the 16+ age group and delivered by schools, colleges, youth clubs and sports centres.

The Youth Sport Trust

The Youth Sport Trust is the key organisation with responsibility for developing school sport. It works with a range of partners including Sport England and Sports Leaders UK. One of its programmes is TOP Sport, which is a Key Stage 2 initiative, with modified equipment suitable for this age group (7–11), as well as lesson plans for teachers linked to NCPE.

The Youth Sport Trust believes in the power of sport to improve the lives of young people. It believes that all youngsters should:
- receive an introduction to PE and sport that links to their developmental needs

- be able to experience and enjoy PE and sport as a result of high-quality teaching, coaching, equipment and resources
- be able to progress along a structured pathway of sporting opportunities (e.g. TOP programmes and extracurricular sporting opportunities via SSCOs)
- develop a sporting lifestyle and foundation for lifelong participation via initiatives such as Step into Sport, School Sport Games and Sky Living for Sport

Tip For the Unit 1 exam you do not need to know the structure of organisations, but it is important that you know how they work in partnership to raise participation levels.

The post-school gap

There is a big drop in participation when young people leave school — the 'post-school gap' — which has concerned the government and sporting institutions for many decades.

Lifelong learning is a government policy that aims to enable people to take part in physical activities that will enrich their lives, and the community, for a long time. Traditionally, the school PE programmes have involved team games, but research suggests that people give up these activities as they get older. In the last decades of the twentieth century, schools began to offer other activities, sometimes using community facilities to promote the opportunities available to young people in their wider community. Activities such as golf, bowls, badminton and swimming are sporting activities that people can continue with for the rest of their lives.

Reasons for the post-school gap	Solutions
Physical education is no longer compulsory	Improve links between schools and clubs so that continued participation is more likely
Young adults have competing leisure interests	Develop knowledge about the need for a healthy lifestyle
Facilities are no longer as accessible or free to use	Offer concessionary rates to young people with a limited disposable income
Traditionally poor links between schools and clubs	Link youth sections at clubs to schools (e.g. share facilities, coaches)

Reasons for government emphasis on PE and school sport

The government believes in the power of PE and sport to improve and enrich people's quality of life, to raise their self-esteem and confidence levels, as well as to provide enjoyment to individuals in society.

Sport is seen as having an important role to play in building stronger, safer communities, strengthening the economy and developing the skills of local people. It also meets the needs of improving the health and fitness of individuals and society in general.

What the examiner will expect you to be able to do

This is a large section of the specification and it requires carefully structured revision of the main topic areas:

- the historical and social factors that have influenced current PE provision (e.g. public schools)
- the development of state PE from the early twentieth century to post-Second World War
- the characteristics of National Curriculum PE (Key Stages 1–4) and its relevance to increasing participation
- the factors affecting school PE provision and the impact it has on a pupil's PE experience
- how school–club links are affecting schools and clubs in providing sport and recreation opportunities for young people
- a number of initiatives (e.g. PESSCL strategy, TOP programmes, SSCOs, Sports colleges, Active Sports) and organisations (e.g. Sport England, Sports Leaders UK, Youth Sport Trust, national governing bodies of sport), and how they are benefiting individuals and communities by raising participation levels

Barriers to participation

There are a number of key terms you need to understand when studying equal opportunities in sport and recreation. Three of these — prejudice, discrimination and stereotyping — are important reasons for inequality, both in the past and at present.

- **Prejudice** means to form an unfavourable opinion of an individual, often based on inadequate facts (e.g. lack of tolerance of people from a specific race or religion).
- **Discrimination** is the unfair treatment of a person, racial group or minority — an action based on prejudice.
- **Stereotyping** is making simplistic generalisations about a group that allows others to categorise them and treat them accordingly.

In Unit 1, four groups are identified (women, ethnic minorities, people with disabilities and lower social classes) and their lack of participation in sport can be linked to a number of factors, including prejudice, discrimination and stereotyping.

Increasing participation in sport is helping to achieve an important aim for local and central government — to decrease exclusion (and therefore increase inclusion) in society. Local and national governments continue to invest resources in sport and recreation schemes to try to create a sense of worth in society in an effort to combat social exclusion.

- **Social exclusion** occurs when certain sections of society are left out of the mainstream; this can happen when people suffer from a range of linked problems (e.g. unemployment, low income and poor housing).

- **Inclusive sport** means that all people have the right to equal opportunities according to their particular needs.

The performance pyramid

The performance pyramid helps to focus discussions about participation.
- The **foundation** level — sometimes called the grass-roots stage of development — is an introduction to physical activity for young children. Basic movement skills and a positive attitude to physical activity are developed from an early age.
- The **participation** level has an emphasis on fun, socialising and formation of friendships. At school this may be through **extra-curricular** activities.
- The **performance** level means county or regional levels of performance, and individuals receive specialist coaching to improve their standard.
- A limited few reach the **excellence** level. Such elite performers strive to represent their country and are fully committed to their sport.

The focus in Unit 1 is on the bottom two levels of the pyramid. Our consideration of various target groups is concerned with widening the base of the pyramid at foundation level and increasing the numbers participating recreationally, that is, at the participation level.

Sport and mass participation

The idea of mass participation in sport is that everyone should have the chance to take part in sport as often as they like and at whatever level they choose. However, the reality does not always match the 'Sport for All' principle of equal opportunities.

Target groups are sections of society identified by Sport England as needing special attention. The aim is to raise participation levels so that they have equality of sporting opportunity. Target groups include ethnic minorities, women, young people (16–24), the elderly, lower social-class groups and people with disabilities.

Under-representation of women in sport

A number of reasons can be given to explain the under-representation of women in sport:
- stereotypical myths (e.g. the belief that physical activity could damage fertility, or that women are not aggressive)
- less media coverage
- fewer role models
- fewer sponsorship opportunities
- lower prize money
- negative effects of school PE programmes (e.g. lack of choice, rules on kit)
- lack of time due to work and family responsibilities
- lack of disposable income
- fewer female coaches and officials

Solutions to gender inequalities

Women's representation in sport is still low in relation to their numbers in society but improvements are being made. Reasons include:

- greater social acceptance of women having jobs and financial independence
- increased media coverage of women's sport
- positive female role models to aspire to
- education to refute stereotypical myths
- more women qualified to coach or officiate in women's (and in some cases men's) sport
- more clubs for women to join and competitions to enter
- the Women's Sports Foundation (see **www.wsf.org.uk**) promotes the benefits of exercise for women and works with other organisations to develop campaigns and policies, such as Sports Coach UK and Women into High Performance Coaching

Race and religion in sport

Britain is a multicultural, multiracial, egalitarian society. Equal opportunities to participate in sport should exist for all racial groups in society. Such equality is not a reality due to many factors, including racism.

You need to understand the following key terms:

- **ethnic groups** — people who have racial, religious or linguistic traits in common
- **racism** — a set of beliefs based on the assumption that races have distinct hereditary characteristics that give some races an intrinsic superiority over others; it may lead to physical or verbal abuse

Racism is illegal but it still exists in society (and therefore sport as a reflection of society) on the basis of colour, language or culture. Racism stems from prejudice linked with the power of one racial group over another. This leads to discrimination, or unfair treatment. For example, teachers might assign students to certain sports or positions on the basis of ascribed ethnic characteristics rather than interests and abilities.

Other causes of under-representation of certain ethnic groups in sports and physical recreation include:

- conflict with religious observances
- a higher value placed on education (less support from family for sports participation)
- racist abuse
- fewer role models (particularly as coaches and managers)
- lower self-esteem and fear of rejection

Possible solutions to racial disadvantage and discrimination include:

- training more ethnic minority sports teachers and coaches, and educating them on the effects of stereotyping
- ensuring there is single-sex provision for Muslim women
- publicising and punishing severely any racist abuse
- organising campaigns against racism in sport
- making more provision in PE programmes for different ethnic preferences, e.g. relaxing kit and showering rules to accommodate cultural norms

Under-representation of people with disabilities in sport

Generally, people with disabilities have a low level of participation in sport. Disability may be physical, sensory or mental in nature, with all of these potentially affecting participation in a negative way. Society continues to discriminate against, and impose barriers on, disabled people's participation in physical activity.

The key terms you need to know are:
- **inclusiveness** — the idea that all people should have their needs, abilities and aspirations recognised, understood and met within a supportive environment
- **integration** — able-bodied and disabled people taking part in the same activity at the same time
- **segregation** — people with disabilities participating separately among themselves

Integration versus segregation

For some disabled individuals, inclusiveness is best realised by integration, while for others segregation may be better.

Potentially, integration has a number of benefits for disabled individuals, such as increasing their self-esteem, breaking down negative stereotypes and helping them to feel more valued in society. However, integration can also affect people with disabilities in negative ways, including safety concerns that have to be addressed and lower self-esteem if they are continually unsuccessful.

Segregation may lead to positive outcomes for the disabled, such as increased success. The negative aspects of segregation include reinforcement of the notion that the disabled are different from the rest of society, which may make them feel less valued and excluded from the mainstream.

Solutions to under-representation of disabled people in sport

Cause	Solution
Negative self-image, lack confidence	Provide opportunities for success
Low income levels	Increase investment in disabled sport to make it more affordable
Poor access to facilities, poor access in and around them	Provide transport to facilities; improve access in and around them
Low levels of media coverage, few role models	Increase media coverage of disabled sport, e.g. Paralympics
Low levels of funding	Increase funding from the National Lottery
Few competitions and clubs	More competitions at all levels; more clubs for the disabled in a wider variety of sports
Myths and stereotypes	Educate people about the myths concerning disabled individuals and challenge inappropriate attitudes

Disability Sport England (**www.dse.org.uk**) is a specialist organisation involved in trying to increase participation among people with disabilities.

For disabled individuals, the benefits of participating in sport include:
- raised levels of confidence and self-esteem
- improved levels of physical skill
- increased health and fitness
- inclusion and integration into society
- more role models to encourage participation
- reducing myths and stereotypes about the disabled

Social class

Social class refers to income, background, social status and education. Playing and watching sport costs money. The more money a person has, the greater the opportunity to take part in or to watch sports.

A three-tier society is still broadly in evidence in the UK today and can be linked to sporting participation as follows:
- upper class — polo, equestrianism and field sports
- middle class — hockey, tennis, golf and rugby union
- working class — football, darts, snooker and rugby league

There is evidence that people with lower socioeconomic status participate less in sport. This is attributed to factors such as cost, lower levels of health and fitness, low self-esteem and lack of opportunities to take up sport or to become role models in positions of responsibility. People from lower socioeconomic backgrounds are more likely to suffer from social exclusion as they have less power, income and self-confidence.

Subsidised provision to encourage participation in local community schemes can help to overcome these barriers, for example Sport Action Zones set up by Sport England in some inner city areas. Such schemes also serve important functions as diversions from crime and general social disorder.

What the examiner will expect you to be able to do
- Understand and define:
  - equal opportunity
  - discrimination
  - stereotyping
  - inclusiveness
  - prejudice
- Identify the barriers to participation for various target groups, including gender, ethnicity, disability and socioeconomic class, and suggest solutions to overcome discrimination and raise participation.

Questions
&
Answers

This section of the guide contains questions that are similar in style to those you can expect to see in the Unit 1 exam. The questions cover all the areas of the specification identified in the Content Guidance section.

Each question is followed by an average or poor response (Candidate A) and an A-grade response (Candidate B).

You should try to answer these questions yourself, so that you can compare your answers with the candidates' responses. In this way, you should be able to identify your strengths and weaknesses in both subject knowledge and exam technique.

All candidate responses are followed by examiner's comments. These are preceded by the icon 𝓮 and indicate where credit is due. In the weaker answers they also point out areas for improvement, specific problems and common errors, such as vagueness, irrelevance and misinterpretation of the question.

Question 1

Health, exercise and fitness

(a) **Identify two components of fitness that are required by a sprint swimmer. Give an example of how one of these components is used in a race.** (3 marks)

(b) **A timed 30 m sprint can be used as a test for power. Discuss whether this test is valid *and* reliable for high jumpers.** (4 marks)

Total: 7 marks

Candidates' answers to Question 1

Candidate A

(a) Speed ✓ and reaction time ✓.

> 🖉 Having correctly identified two fitness components required by a sprint swimmer, Candidate A forgets to say how one of these components is used during a race. Always read the question carefully and check your answer. Look at the number of marks available — this indicates the number of points you need to make. Candidate A scores 2 marks.

Candidate B

(a) Speed ✓ and power ✓. Power is needed to get off the blocks with as much force as possible ✓.

> 🖉 Candidate B correctly names two relevant fitness components required by a sprint swimmer and then says when one of these is important in a race. Always choose the fitness components that are most relevant to the sporting activity asked for. Candidate B scores all 3 marks.

Candidate A

(b) A high jumper needs to jump up into the air. The 30 m sprint test does not test for this, so it is not valid ✓. However, the high jumper does need speed and strength and these are tested by the 30 m sprint ✓, so it is reliable.

> 🖉 Candidate A gives reasons why the 30 m sprint test is not valid. However, no explanation has been given of reliability, despite using the term in the second part of the answer. Make sure you are clear about the differences between validity and reliability. Candidate A scores 2 marks.

Candidate B

(b) A valid test should measure exactly what it sets out to do. The 30 m sprint involves strength and speed, which are valid for a high jumper ✓. However, it is not sport-specific because it does not reflect the high-jumping action ✓. Reliability concerns the accuracy of the test. This test is repeatable ✓ but the performer must be motivated to complete the test ✓.

🖉 This is a top-level answer, which scores full marks. The candidate clarifies validity and reliability, which makes it easier to explain the relevance of the test to the high jumper. There are 4 marks available and four correct points are made.

■ ■ ■

Question 2

Nutrition

(a) Eating a diet with sufficient calcium and iron has physiological benefits for an athlete. State the importance of these two minerals for the athlete. (3 marks)

(b) In what ways should the diet of a long-distance runner be different from that of a weightlifter? Give reasons for your answer. (3 marks)

Total: 6 marks

Candidates' answers to Question 2

Candidate A

(a) Calcium is good for bones ✓ and iron helps produce haemoglobin ✓.

🖉 The physiological benefits of calcium and iron are stated correctly but this information has not been related to the athlete. Weaker candidates often forget to apply their knowledge. Candidate A scores 2 marks.

Candidate B

(a) Calcium is good for bones ✓ and is important for nerve transmission and muscle contraction ✓. Iron is beneficial in the production of red blood cells ✓ and this will improve the transportation of oxygen in the athlete ✓.

🖉 Candidate B explains the benefits of calcium and iron and then relates their importance to the athlete. Four points are made but the maximum score allowed is 3 marks. Some questions do not specifically ask for definitions but including them or giving an explanation can score marks. This is a thorough answer, which scores the full 3 marks.

Candidate A

(b) A long-distance runner requires more carbohydrates ✓ and a weightlifter needs more protein ✓.

🖉 This answer scores 2 marks. A common mistake is made here. Candidates often answer the first part of a question and forget to answer the second part.

Always check your work when you have finished to see if you have missed any answers.

Candidate B

(b) A long-distance runner uses carbohydrate ✓ for energy ✓ and a weightlifter uses protein ✓ for muscle growth ✓.

> 💡 Again, Candidate B has answered both parts of the question correctly and has made more points than there are marks allowed. Candidate B scores 3 marks.

■ ■ ■

Question 3
Pulmonary function

(a) During exercise, the oxyhaemoglobin curve shifts to the right. Explain the causes of this change and identify the effect this has on oxygen delivery to the muscles. (4 marks)

(b) The breathing characteristics of games players alter during performance. The table shows the percentages of oxygen and carbon dioxide breathed out during exercise compared with at rest.

	Inhaled air	Exhaled air (quiet breathing)	Exhaled air (exercise)
Oxygen (%)	21	17	15
Carbon dioxide (%)	0.04	4	6

Use information from the table to describe the effects of exercise on gas exchange in the lungs. Suggest why these changes occur. (3 marks)

(c) Explain the causes of the increase in breathing rate experienced during exercise. (4 marks)

Total: 11 marks

Candidates' answers to Question 3

Candidate A

(a) The curve shifts to the right because the muscles need more oxygen. This is called the Bohr shift ✓.

> 💡 Candidate A scores 1 mark out of 4. This question appears regularly in some format and many candidates have difficulty in answering it. Try to learn two or three causes, and remember that the curve shifts to the right not because the muscles

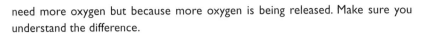

need more oxygen but because more oxygen is being released. Make sure you understand the difference.

Candidate B

(a) When the curve moves to the right it is called the Bohr shift ✓. It is caused by an increase in blood temperature ✓ and carbon dioxide ✓. This means that more oxygen is released to the muscle more quickly ✓.

🖉 This is a clear, logically structured answer that scores full marks. An increase in the acidity of blood is another cause that could be given.

Candidate A

(b) From the table there is more oxygen consumed. This is because it is needed for energy ✓.

🖉 This question requires candidates to look at the whole table, so an answer that mentions just one gas will automatically lose 1 mark. The candidate should also have referred to carbon dioxide. The fact that Candidate A has only mentioned oxygen affects the second part of the answer too, and a second mark is lost. Candidate A scores 1 mark only.

Candidate B

(b) From the table it can be seen that less oxygen and more carbon dioxide is exhaled during exercise than during quiet breathing ✓. This is because oxygen is used for energy in the working muscles during exercise ✓. Carbon dioxide is a waste product of aerobic respiration ✓.

🖉 This response is detailed and covers all parts of the question. When a table is presented in a question, make sure that you refer to it comprehensively. Candidate B scores all 3 marks.

Candidate A

(c) During exercise there is an increase in carbon dioxide in the blood ✓. As a result impulses are sent to the medulla ✓ and this sends impulses to the lungs to increase breathing rate.

🖉 With a little more detail, this answer could have gained full marks. Candidate A identifies an increase in carbon dioxide but does not say that this is detected by chemoreceptors. Saying that an impulse goes to the lungs is almost correct, but you should know exactly where the impulses are sent, i.e. to the respiratory muscles. Always give as much detail as possible. Candidate A scores 2 marks.

Candidate B

(c) There is an increase in the production of carbon dioxide ✓ and therefore blood acidity ✓. This is detected by chemoreceptors ✓. Impulses are sent to the respiratory centre located in the medulla ✓, which in turn sends impulses to the diaphragm and to the external intercostals ✓.

🖉 Candidate B makes five correct points, one more than the number of marks allocated. Generally, with questions that do not specify a particular number, it is good exam technique to look at the mark allocation and make more points than there are marks available, in an attempt to ensure the possibility of a maximum mark. However, if a question specifies a number (e.g. 'Give two…'), only the first two answers will be marked. Candidate B scores all 4 marks.

■ ■ ■

Question 4
Transport of blood gases

Explain how blood flow is redistributed to the working muscles. (3 marks)

Total: 3 marks

Candidates' answers to Question 4

Candidate A
Blood needs to be redistributed to the working muscles because they need more oxygen for energy.

> ⟲ This answer fails to score. A common error made by candidates with this question is to explain *why* blood is redistributed to the working muscles and not *how*. Always read the question carefully and highlight the words that indicate the requirements of the question.

Candidate B
An increase in carbon dioxide ✓ is detected by chemoreceptors ✓. An impulse is then sent to the medulla ✓ and vasodilation in the arterioles leading to the working muscles occurs ✓. Vasoconstriction also takes place in the arterioles leading to the non-essential organs ✓.

> ⟲ Candidate B scores the maximum 3 marks. This is a detailed answer and correct terminology is used, but most importantly the candidate has explained *how* redistribution takes place.

■ ■ ■

Question 5
Cardiac function

(a) Heart rate and stroke volume both increase during exercise. What causes the increase in stroke volume? (2 marks)

(b) The heart rate increases before and during exercise and then decreases after exercise. Explain how these changes in heart rate occur. (4 marks)

Total: 6 marks

Candidates' answers to Question 5

Candidate A
(a) An increase in stroke volume is caused by an increase in venous return ✓, which means more blood can be pumped out of the heart.

> 🖉 Only 1 mark can be awarded because the mark scheme classes these two points made as similar — one is the result of the other. If the candidate had made more points than the number of marks allocated, then both marks might have been gained.

Candidate B
(a) An increase in stroke volume is caused by an increase in the strength of contraction of the heart ✓. This means more blood can be ejected by the heart ✓.

> 🖉 This answer gives two correct responses and scores both marks. The candidate could have said that an increase in stroke volume is also caused by adrenaline and by nervous control.

Candidate A
(b) Adrenaline causes an increase in heart rate before exercise ✓. During exercise, receptors detect changes, such as an increase in carbon dioxide ✓. They send impulses to the brain, which increase heart rate.

> 🖉 Candidate A does not specify chemoreceptors and loses a mark. 'Brain' is too vague to score — the candidate should have mentioned the cardiac centre. Similarly, the SA node should have been cited, rather than simply 'heart'. The lack of detail in this mediocre answer means that Candidate A scores only 2 marks.

Candidate B
(b) An increase in heart rate prior to exercise is due to adrenaline ✓. During exercise, there is an increase in carbon dioxide ✓ and therefore an increase in acidity ✓. This is detected by chemoreceptors ✓ and an impulse is sent to the cardiac centre ✓. This in turn sends an impulse to the SA node to increase heart rate ✓. After exercise, the parasympathetic nervous system decreases heart rate ✓.

> 🖉 This comprehensive answer easily scores all 4 marks. The candidate has covered several more points than there are marks available. This is good exam technique if the nature of the question allows you to do this.

■ ■ ■

Question 6

Analysis of movement

(a) The preparation phase for the jump shown in the diagram involves a downward movement.

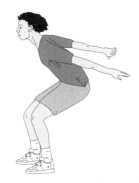

Complete the table to show the types of joint and joint action involved, the main agonist and the type of contraction that occurs during this downward phase.

(9 marks)

	Type of joint	Joint action	Agonist	Type of contraction
Hip		Flexion		
Knee				Eccentric
Ankle	Hinge			

(b)

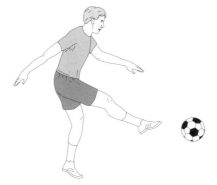

With reference to the knee joint of the kicking leg of the footballer:
(i) Name the articulating bones. (1 mark)
(ii) At the moment leading up to impact, what joint action is taking place at the knee joint and what is the name of the agonist causing this action? (2 marks)

(c) **Name the lever system that operates at the elbow during flexion.**
Sketch and label a diagram to show this type of lever. (3 marks)

Total: 15 marks

Candidates' answers to Question 6

Candidate A

(a)

	Type of joint	Joint action	Agonist	Type of contraction
Hip	Ball and socket ✓	Flexion	Hamstrings ✓	Isotonic ✓
Knee	Hinge ✓	Flexion ✓	Quads	Eccentric
Ankle	Hinge	Flexion	Gastrocnemius ✓	Isotonic

    This response lacks sufficient detail. You must be specific. The movement in the
ankle joint is *dorsiflexion* — flexion will not score the mark. Abbreviating muscle
names will also prevent a mark being awarded — for example, 'quads' is not an
acceptable answer, whereas 'quadriceps' is. Similarly, you need to be specific about
the type of muscle contraction. By using 'isotonic' twice, Candidate A is limited to
1 mark. To gain both the available marks for contraction, the candidate should have
given the *type* of isotonic contraction, i.e. eccentric. Candidate A scores 6 of the
9 marks available.

Candidate B

(a)

	Type of joint	Joint action	Agonist	Type of contraction
Hip	Ball and socket ✓	Flexion	Hamstrings ✓	Eccentric ✓
Knee	Hinge ✓	Flexion ✓	Quadriceps ✓	Eccentric
Ankle	Hinge	Dorsiflexion ✓	Gastrocnemius ✓	Eccentric ✓

    There is 1 mark available for each correct answer in the table. The candidate has
correctly identified the types of joint, joint action, the muscles involved and the
types of contraction and scores all 9 marks.

Candidate A

(b) (i) Femur and fibula.

  (ii) The movement is extension ✓ and the agonists are the hamstrings.

    One common mistake candidates make is to name the fibula as one of the artic-
ulating bones of the knee joint. This bone actually stops before it reaches the knee.
Both bones need to be correctly identified to score the mark. Candidates also
often confuse the movement produced by the hamstrings and the quadriceps. This
is an easy mark lost. With more revision, Candidate A would have remembered that
the hamstrings flex the knee and the quadriceps extend the knee. Candidate A
scores 1 mark.

Candidate B

(b) (i) Femur and tibia ✓.

(ii) The joint action is extension ✓ and the agonist is the quadriceps ✓.

> 🖉 This is a top-level answer. All the bones, movement and muscles are correctly identified. Thorough revision of the sporting actions required by the specification will ensure success. Candidate B scores all 3 marks.

Candidate A

(c) This is a third-order lever ✓.

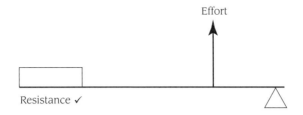

> 🖉 The candidate clearly knows the correct answer but has omitted to label the fulcrum. This means that a mark is lost. Make sure you check all your answers, so that you do not lose easy marks. Candidate A scores 2 marks.

Candidate B

(c) This is a third-order lever ✓.

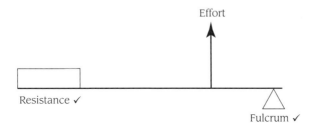

> 🖉 The type of lever is correctly identified and the diagram is fully labelled. Candidate B scores 3 marks.

■ ■ ■

Question 7

Application of theory to a practical situation

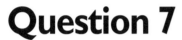 In Section B there is an extended question. Here you need to express your answer clearly and concisely but at the same time demonstrate a range and depth of knowledge. Spelling, punctuation and grammar are important, as is the use of technical language. This question is worth 12 marks and you need to give a balanced answer from both exercise physiology and skill acquisition to get into the top mark band.

(a) Identify and define three types of fitness that are important for a hockey player and offer some nutritional advice to hockey players that will help them to adopt a balanced diet suitable for their sport.

(b) As a hockey coach you can present skills to performers in different ways. Critically evaluate the whole, whole–part–whole and progressive part methods of practising hockey skills.

Candidates' answers to Question 7

Candidate A

(a) The components of fitness a hockey player needs are coordination, speed, reaction time and power. They should be eating lots of carbohydrates ✓ for energy ✓ and no fats, as they do not want to be overweight. It is also important that they drink lots of water so that they do not dehydrate.

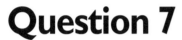 Candidates can choose any three from agility, speed, flexibility, coordination and power. The candidate correctly identifies coordination and speed but loses potential marks because reaction time is wrong. Power is correct but it will not be marked because the question asks for *three* components and the examiner may only mark the first three answers given. The answer to the second part of the question makes two points, but the other types of food should have been discussed. Candidate A scores 2 marks, which places him/her in the bottom band for this part of the question.

Candidate B

(a) Three components of fitness that are important in hockey are agility, speed and power ✓. Agility is the ability to change direction quickly ✓. Speed is how fast a specific distance can be covered ✓ and power is a combination of strength and speed ✓. A balanced diet for a hockey player would consist of 10–15% protein, 20–25% fat and 60–75% carbohydrate ✓. A high percentage of carbohydrates should be consumed because they are a high-energy food ✓. Fats provide energy for low-intensity exercise ✓ and proteins are used for tissue growth ✓. Minerals are useful too, calcium for strong bones and iron helps form haemoglobin ✓. Consuming sports drinks such as Lucozade can boost glucose levels before competition ✓.

🖉 Candidate B has made a wide variety of points. The answer is concise, well explained and uses technical language. Candidate B makes the required number of points to be placed at the top of the top band for this part of the question.

Candidate A

(b) The whole method means practising the skill as a whole. For example, a hit in hockey ✓ has to be practised as a whole. The whole–part–whole method means doing a skill as a whole, focusing on one bit of it, then doing it as a whole again. This might be for a skill like a penalty flick ✓. You do the whole routine and then practise one bit, like the placement of the stick in relation to the ball and the feet, then do the whole routine again. The progressive part method means you do all the parts of the skill and put them together at the end. In a trampoline routine this would mean, for example, practising the seat drop, then the back drop and then the somersault individually and then once they are all perfect put them together as one.

🖉 Candidate A has attempted to address all three parts of the question. In the description of the whole and whole–part–whole methods, using the word 'whole' is repeating the question. The candidate should use alternative wording, such as 'in its entirety' or 'in full'. The example of a hit is correct but the candidate has not stated why it should be practised as a whole. The example of a penalty flick is correct for the whole–part–whole method but the description and reasons for using this method are vague. The candidate has made a common mistake in the description of the progressive part method: stating that each part should be learned and then practised together at the end is not correct. Candidates often find it difficult to think of a relevant example, so choose a different sport such as a trampoline routine. Candidate A is again in the bottom band of marks, as few relevant points are made.

Candidate B

(b) Whole practice is good for skills that are high ✓ in organisation and cannot be broken down into their subroutines. An example is a hit in hockey ✓. The performer has to practise these skills in their entirety ✓, as the subroutines are too difficult to separate. This is a good method for developing kinaesthesis ✓ and it is not time-consuming ✓. However, as the performer is shown the whole skill, he/she may experience information overload ✓. This is a good method for autonomous ✓ performers.

The whole–part–whole method is a better method as it allows the performer to experience the whole skill but also allows him/her to work on weaknesses ✓. For example, with the penalty corner, the coach will allow the team to perform the whole routine and may notice that the positioning of the players is weak ✓.

The coach will look at this part of the penalty corner, offer advice, then try the whole skill again. This method takes longer ✓ than the whole method.

The final method is the progressive part method. This is also for skills that are low in organisation and can be broken down into subroutines, or for serial skills that are made up of discrete skills run in order. It takes a vast amount of time ✓ to use this method, but the performer will be motivated by being successful in each of the parts. Using the penalty corner as an example, you would learn the pushout first and practise it. Then you would learn and practise the stop and put these two steps together. You would then learn the shot at goal and add that until the whole skill is performed ✓.

> 🖉 This is a detailed answer showing comprehensive knowledge of the topic area. Candidate B has given some advantages and disadvantages of each method and has linked theory to practice several times. The candidate has linked the question to classification of skill and phases of learning, showing knowledge of other areas of the specification. It is written in continuous prose and has technical vocabulary throughout, showing good written communication. The examiner would have no difficulty in awarding full marks and placing this answer in the top band.

■ ■ ■

Question 8

Classification of skills

(a) Using practical examples, explain the pacing continuum. (4 marks)

(b) Classify the front crawl on the continuity and muscular involvement continua and justify your answer. (2 marks)

Total: 6 marks

Candidates' answers to Question 8

Candidate A

(a) A self-paced skill is when you decide on the pace of the skill. For example, a tennis serve. An externally paced skill is when your opponent or team-mates control the pace of the skill.

> 🖉 This is a weak answer. The candidate repeats the question by using the word pace. In order to score, you must use an alternative word such as rate, timing or speed. A tennis serve is a self-paced skill but the description is too vague to be given credit. Candidate A fails to score.

Candidate B

(a) The pacing continuum describes who controls the timing and speed of the skill ✓. A cartwheel is a self-paced skill ✓ because the performer dictates when and how fast the skill is performed ✓. Receiving a pass in rugby is an externally paced skill ✓ because the performer cannot control how fast the ball is thrown ✓ to him/her.

> 🖉 This is an excellent answer. It explains the continuum and then goes on to describe the extremes of the continuum. Practical examples are given for the extremes and these are very clear, ensuring the examiner will give credit. Candidate B scores 4 marks.

Candidate A

(b) Front crawl is continuous ✓ and gross.

> 🖉 Candidate A has correctly classified the skill but has not justified the reasons for this. In this case, it is usual for a sub-maximum mark to be placed on the answer. Without justification, only 1 mark can be awarded.

Candidate B

(b) The front crawl is a continuous skill because it has no clear start and stop ✓. It is a cycle where the end of one stroke is the beginning of the next. It is also a gross skill because it uses a lot of large ✓ muscles in the body.

> 🖉 This is an excellent answer that addresses both parts of the question. The easiest way to justify anything is to use the word 'because'. Candidate B scores 2 marks.

■ ■ ■

Question 9

Abilities

(a) Give two characteristics of ability. (2 marks)

(b) What are gross motor ability and psychomotor ability? Use practical examples to illustrate your answer. (4 marks)

Total: 6 marks

Candidates' answers to Question 9

Candidate A

(a) Abilities are genetically determined ✓. We get our abilities from our parents. They are stable.

The question specifies the number of answers required, so only the first two points will be marked, in this case, genetically determined and from our parents. Although both of these are correct, they are similar, and therefore only worthy of 1 mark. The next point is correct but cannot be marked. Make sure your answers are clearly separate. Candidate A scores 1 mark.

Candidate B

(a) Abilities are the building blocks of skills ✓. Abilities are stable ✓.

Candidate B has answered succinctly and correctly, and scores both marks.

Candidate A

(b) Gross motor ability is using our innate abilities to perform large muscle group movements ✓. For example, strength. Psychomotor ability is reaction time.

This is a weak answer. The description of gross motor ability is well written and scores a mark, but the example is vague. The candidate should have stated that strength is used when performing a power lift, for example. Identifying a motor ability alone is not enough. Reaction time is a psychomotor ability but there is no clear explanation. Candidate A scores 1 mark.

Candidate B

(b) Gross motor ability is a performer's natural ability when performing large muscle group movements ✓. For example, using your stamina in a marathon ✓. Psychomotor ability is about linking the mind with the body. It is when a performer processes information quickly and puts their decisions into action ✓. For example, when you judge how fast a football is being passed to you and you move closer towards it as it is slow ✓.

This is a good attempt to answer a question that candidates often have difficulty with. The examples are clear enough to gain marks. In some cases, this question would be worth only 2 marks in total, so here both the explanation and the example must be credit worthy. Candidate B scores 4 marks.

■ ■ ■

Question 10
Stages of learning

(a) Using practical examples, describe the three phases of learning.　　(6 marks)

(b) What are the functions of feedback?　　(3 marks)

Total: 9 marks

Candidates' answers to Question 10

Candidate A

(a) Phase one is the beginners. They are slow and always have to look down and focus on the ball in basketball ✓. Phase two is intermediates. They can look up to pass and make fewer mistakes. Phase three is the experts. They are smooth when passing ✓.

> This 6-mark question requires much more detail. The candidate has offered some correct descriptions and examples but much more time should be given to this relatively straightforward question. Candidate A scores 2 marks.

Candidate B

(a) The first phase of learning is the cognitive phase. Movements are jerky ✓ and the learner makes a lot of mistakes ✓. When dribbling, a hockey player will start and stop and lose the ball several times.

In the second stage the hockey player will start to notice that he is making mistakes and change ✓ his body or grip to rectify it. He will begin to develop kinaesthesis ✓ and know how dribbling should feel.

In the final stage the performers are known as autonomous. They are experts. When dribbling they are fluent ✓ and make few mistakes. They can focus on their position on the field and where to run to next ✓.

> This answer shows great exam technique and scores the full 6 marks. The candidate has given clear examples throughout. By using the same example, the three phases are clearly distinguished. The candidate has not identified the second phase as the associative phase, but the question doesn't ask for this and therefore full marks can be awarded.

Candidate A

(b) Intrinsic feedback comes from within. Extrinsic feedback comes from an outside source. Knowledge of performance tells you the technical information about your performance.

> This answer is totally irrelevant and fails to score. This is a common problem when candidates do not read the question properly. Candidate A has answered a question about *types* of feedback rather than *functions* of feedback. Make sure you read the question carefully and highlight the main words.

Candidate B

(b) Feedback tells you what you are doing correctly ✓ and detects errors ✓. If a coach tells you that you are doing something correctly, it raises your confidence ✓ and motivates ✓ you. For example, when you perform a tennis serve correctly, the coach will say, 'Well done, good speed in the serve'.

This is an excellent answer, which scores the full 3 marks. It gives more points than there are marks available and gives a practical example although it is not asked for in the question. This is good practice. There is some repetition regarding feedback informing you of correct actions — this will not gain further marks but the candidate will not be penalised.

■ ■ ■

Question 11

Information processing

(a) **What is selective attention and why is it important for the short-term memory?** (3 marks)

(b) **Define reaction time, movement time and response time, using practical examples.** (3 marks)

(c) **One way of outwitting opponents is by 'selling a dummy'. Explain this in terms of the psychological refractory period.** (5 marks)

Total: 11 marks

Candidates' answers to Question 11

Candidate A

(a) Selective attention is when a performer blocks out the crowd and focuses on just the ball ✓. It is important because the short-term memory can only hold between five and nine items ✓. The short-term memory only lasts between 15 and 30 seconds.

Both parts of the question have been addressed. Often candidates fail to do so with such questions. The candidate has not given a clear definition of selective attention, but the attempt through an example would probably gain a benefit of the doubt (BOD) mark. The candidate has given clear reasons for the importance of selective attention to the short-term memory. The points about the amount and length of storage are both correct but are the same points on the mark scheme and therefore gain only 1 mark. Candidate A scores 2 marks.

Candidate B

(a) Selective attention is filtering the relevant information from the irrelevant ✓. For example, in rugby the player will focus on the ball and the incoming tackler rather than the rest of the players on the pitch and the spectators. The short-term memory has a limited capacity of five to nine items ✓ and therefore selective attention prevents information overload as it filters away the irrelevant items such as the crowd ✓.

This is a good answer where both parts of the question have been addressed. Selective attention has been clearly defined and reinforced with an example. Only 1 mark is available for this part of the question, but this shows the examiner that the candidate has the relevant knowledge and can apply it to a practical situation. The importance of selective attention is clearly discussed, again with the help of a practical example. Candidate B scores all 3 marks.

Candidate A

(b) Reaction time is from when the stimulus is first seen or heard to when you start to move, e.g. from when the swimmer hears the starter's beep to when they dive in ✓. Movement time is the time of the whole movement, e.g. performing the dive. Response time is reaction time plus movement time.

The candidate attempts to address all three parts of the question. Although a little vague, credit would be awarded for the answer about reaction time. The answer about movement time repeats the question and the example is vague. Response time is a combination of reaction and movement time — however, no practical example is given.

Candidate B

(b) Reaction time is the time from the onset of the stimulus to the onset of the response. For example, in the 100 m, this is from the gun being shot to the sprinter pushing on the blocks ✓. Movement time is the onset of the response to the completion of the task. In the 100 m, this will be from when the performer pushes on the blocks to when he/she crosses the finish line ✓. Response time is from the onset of the stimulus to the completion of the task. In the 100 m, this will be from the gun shot to the sprinter crossing the line ✓.

Candidate B scores 3 marks for this succinct and word-perfect answer. The candidate has addressed all three parts of the question and given a clear practical example for each. The sprint start example is usually the easiest to describe.

Candidate A

(c) When you 'sell a dummy', you go one way then change your mind and go the other. This is the psychological refractory period.

This answer is far too brief for a 5-mark question. It doesn't say what the psychological refractory period is — it just repeats the question. Although it describes a dummy, it does not expand on this in terms of linking the theory with the practical. Candidate A fails to score.

Candidate B

(c) The psychological refractory period occurs when a second stimulus arrives before the first stimulus has been processed ✓. This is because the brain can only process one item at a time and causes the performer to freeze. In rugby, the first stimulus from the attacker would be to pretend to pass to the right ✓. The first response from the defender would be to follow ✓ the pass. The attacker would then

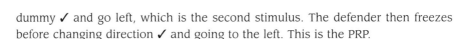

dummy ✓ and go left, which is the second stimulus. The defender then freezes before changing direction ✓ and going to the left. This is the PRP.

🖉 This is an excellent answer. The candidate has answered the question fully and given a correct practical example. Candidate B scores 5 marks out of 5.

■ ■ ■

Question 12
The nature and characteristics of physical activities

(a) **PE teachers aim to develop their pupils' knowledge and values. Identify values and benefits to be gained from a positive school PE experience.** (4 marks)

(b) **Play is often considered to be an educational experience. What can children learn through play?** (4 marks)

(c) **What are the main characteristics of sport?** (5 marks)

(d) **Apart from games, identify all other areas of activity within the National Curriculum for PE.** (3 marks)

Total: 16 marks

Candidates' answers to Question 12

Candidate A
(a) Having a positive PE experience may encourage you to take up sport when you are older ✓. This can improve your health and general wellbeing ✓. Having a good experience can also help encourage young children to participate in sport.

🖉 The first two sentences earn marks as they are linked to the 'preparation for leisure' and 'improved health' values of PE. The final sentence is vague and too similar to the first point to earn another mark. The answer is too brief and lacks a range of different points. Candidate A scores 2 marks.

Candidate B
(a) A positive PE experience can lead to:
- the development of physical skills ✓
- health benefits ✓
- knowledge of the rules of a sport ✓
- help in getting a job or career in sport ✓
- an improvement in self-confidence ✓
- making friends and improving social skills ✓

✍ All six points are worth a mark. This answer is written in an examiner-friendly way with a brief introduction and the key points listed as bullets. More points have been made than there are marks available, to try to ensure full marks are earned. Candidate B scores all 4 marks.

Candidate A

(b) Children can learn how to play fairly and respect the rules of a game ✓. They can learn about sportsmanship and accepting defeat. They also learn basic skills, such as throwing and catching ✓.

✍ This is an example of an answer that is factually correct but focuses too much on one point — fair play. The second sentence repeats the first, so a mark cannot be awarded. Without the practical example, the 'basic skills' point may not have been awarded because 'skills' could relate to physical, mental or social development. Candidate A scores 2 marks.

Candidate B

(b) • Children can learn how to interact with others ✓.
• They learn fundamental motor skills by playing with such things as balls ✓.
• They learn cognitive skills by problem solving ✓.
• They learn how to cooperate and work together as a team ✓.
• When making up their own games, they learn creative skills ✓.
• They learn how to play safely ✓.

✍ All six points are relevant and answer the question in a clear and succinct manner. Use of practical examples is further evidence of good exam practice, as is the fact that more points have been made than there are marks available. Candidate B scores all 4 marks.

Candidate A

(c) Sport is played professionally at high levels ✓. People such as Wayne Rooney earn lots of money from playing football for a living. He is a role model. I want to be like him because he plays at a high level for my favourite club. The skills he produces on the pitch are fantastic, which again makes me want to be like him ✓.

✍ Although the use of practical examples to illustrate your understanding is to be encouraged, in this case too much focus on one person has limited the number of marks gained. Repeating the point about a professional playing for high rewards at a high level means only 1 mark can be gained because the characteristics are so similar. Reference to high skill levels gains a second mark. A variety of points should have been made in answer to this relatively simple question. Candidate A scores only 2 of the 5 available marks.

Candidate B

(c) Sport has a number of characteristics, such as:
• competitiveness and the will to win ✓
• rules ✓
• high fitness demands ✓

- governing bodies (e.g. the LTA) ✓
- use of specialist equipment ✓
- officials that make decisions

🖉 Just enough relevant points are made to gain maximum marks. The final point cannot be awarded a mark because it repeats the point about 'rules'. It would have been a good idea to make one or two more points, in case of vagueness or more repetition. Missing out on maximum marks on relatively easy questions can make a significant difference to the final grade achieved. Unless a specific number is asked for in the question, always make more points than there are marks available. Candidate B scores all 5 marks.

Candidate A

(d) In my PE lessons I play a lot of sport and different games such as football, cricket and tennis. I also do lots of running.

🖉 This answer is a vague attempt to earn a few marks despite a lack of knowledge of the areas of activity defined in the National Curriculum PE. The candidate should have highlighted or underlined 'Apart from games' in the question before starting to answer. This would have ensured that games were not included in the answer. If the final point about running had been linked to athletics, then it would have earned a mark. Candidate A fails to score.

Candidate B

(d) National Curriculum PE has a number of different areas of activity:
- gymnastics and dance ✓
- swimming and athletics ✓
- outdoor and adventurous activities ✓

🖉 This is an examiner-friendly way of giving an answer in a relevant, clear and succinct manner. All areas of activity identified are correct, for full marks.

■ ■ ■

Question 13
Historical developments in sport and PE

(a) The physical activities offered by state elementary schools changed during the first half of the twentieth century. Describe and explain these changes. *(7 marks)*

(b) Increasing participation in physical activity within a community is considered a positive act in today's egalitarian society. How do the reasons for increasing participation differ between *local authority* run clubs and *voluntary* clubs? *(4 marks)*

(c) TOP Sport in England is an example of a primary school initiative.
Describe TOP Sport.   (4 marks)

                                                          Total: 15 marks

Candidates' answers to Question 13

Candidate A

(a) In the late nineteenth and early twentieth centuries there was a focus on drill (mainly military) ✓. As the twentieth century began, a more therapeutic approach to drill was introduced ✓. There was also recognition of different ages and sexes of children ✓. Following the Second World War, facilities were improved ✓ and a more child-centred approach was taken to teaching PE ✓.

> 🖉 One part of the question — a description of changes to state PE — has been answered well and earns 4 marks. The final point would receive a mark, had the sub-maximum 4 marks not already been achieved. However, there is no *explanation* of these developments, as required by the question.

Candidate B

(a) Military drill was initially taught to boys only ✓ as preparation for their military service ✓ and also to improve health and fitness ✓. In the early twentieth century, a more therapeutic approach, based on the Swedish system of drill, was introduced ✓. This was due to more emphasis being placed on children having fun ✓. As the twentieth century progressed there was more use of apparatus in schools ✓ and teachers were able to use their own initiative to teach ✓.

> 🖉 This answer is made in a chronologically correct manner and includes relevant points that describe and explain developments in state PE in the early twentieth century. Candidate B scores all 7 marks.

Candidate A

(b) Private-sector clubs, such as David Lloyd fitness centres, provide top-level facilities but can cost a lot of money. Public-sector clubs, such as local authority leisure centres, are cheaper but facilities are not as good. Voluntary-sector clubs, such as my hockey club, aim to provide good facilities to get more members ✓.

> 🖉 This answer has a clear structure and is quite well written, but unfortunately *it does not answer the question set*. It is the start of an analysis of the differences between public, private and voluntary sectors, which focuses too much on facilities and does not relate to reasons for increasing participation. Candidate A scores only 1 mark.

Candidate B

(b) Local authorities want to increase participation to improve the health of individuals ✓ and, therefore, to create a healthier society ✓. There are often benefits to the community. Voluntary clubs want to attract more members ✓ so they have a better chance of winning competitions ✓.

> 🖉 This is a succinct, relevant answer. Both parts of the question are answered, producing a balanced response that earns the maximum 4 marks. With the relatively limited time available in the unit test, it is this type of concise answer that is needed to do well.

Candidate A

(c) TOP Sport is a series of initiatives for children aged from 18 months to 18 years. These range from TOP Tots to TOP Sportsability. They aim to develop skills and fitness through schooling. As the schemes increase, more analysis and coaching becomes involved.

> 🖉 The points made are irrelevant and vague. The question requires a description of TOP Sport, which is one of the TOPS programmes. This should be the focus of the answer. However, Candidate A focuses on describing the range of TOPS programmes available. To make sure that you answer the question set, it might help to highlight key words or phrases in the question before starting to write your answer. Candidate A does not score.

Candidate B

(c) TOP Sport is supported and developed by the Youth Sport Trust ✓. It is designed to support teachers in their delivery of National Curriculum PE ✓ to 7–11-year-olds ✓. Training is provided for teachers to deliver TOP Sport ✓. Bags containing adapted sports-related equipment ✓ are given to teachers to help them deliver TOP Sport. Teaching cards with lesson ideas on them are also provided ✓.

> 🖉 Candidate B has answered the question set and included many relevant points on TOP Sport. More correct points are made than the maximum mark available, which is good exam practice. Candidate B scores all 4 marks.

■ ■ ■

Question 14

Historical and social influences on modern-day sport

(a) How might a person's ethnic background influence his/her participation in physical activity? (4 marks)

(b) Apart from 'adaptations', in what other ways can the participation of people with disabilities be increased? (3 marks)

(c) What social and economic barriers do women face today when attempting to participate in sport or physical activity? (4 marks)

Total: 11 marks

Candidates' answers to Question 14

Candidate A

(a) Ethnic background links to race. Race links to the colour of a person's skin. If you are from an ethnic minority group, you may take part less in sport because you may fear rejection by a sports club ✓ and have low self-esteem. This fear may be due to physical threats ✓ and abuse. Racial discrimination can lower participation levels.

> 🖉 This answer illustrates how a candidate can focus too much on a particular point or two. Though these are explained very well, repeating the same point does not earn marks. To gain more marks, the answer needs to cover a range of different points. Candidate A scores 2 marks.

Candidate B

(a) People's ethnic background influences their involvement in physical activity, because racial discrimination may lower participation ✓. There may be fewer role models in certain sports ✓ but more in others to encourage participation. Higher values placed on education as opposed to sport may limit participation ✓. Lower levels of self-esteem may put off ethnic minorities from taking part in sport ✓.

> 🖉 Four relevant and sufficiently varied points are made to earn full marks.

Candidate A

(b) Disabled people often struggle to get around leisure centres ✓. They need lifts and ramps to help improve this situation. If television gave more time to disabled sport, it might help increase participation as more role models might be created ✓.

> 🖉 This answer addresses the question set and makes relevant points backed up with examples. All it lacks is a sufficient range of points to earn full marks. Candidate A scores 2 marks.

Candidate B

(b) Participation by disabled people in sport could be increased by providing special times for them at leisure centres ✓. More clubs could be set up for them to join ✓, with specialist coaching provided ✓. If more media coverage was given, for example of the Paralympics, it might increase participation by the disabled ✓.

> 🖉 Candidate B scores all 3 marks. This is an excellent answer, which contains four relevant points to try to ensure maximum marks are gained.

Candidate A

(c) Women still have to look after children more than men ✓. Many sports are seen as too strenuous for women to take part in ✓. Myths and stereotypes still exist about what women can do.

> 🖉 This answer is a little too brief and focuses purely on 'social' factors. In answer to a 'what' question, bullet point lists of social and economic factors linked to women's lack of participation in physical activity would suffice. No specific number of points

is asked for, so relevant educated guesses could be made in an effort to gain more marks. Candidate A scores 2 of the 4 available marks.

Candidate B

(c) • Sexual discrimination still exists in society today ✓.
  • Many males see sport as their preserve ✓.
  • Women tend to have jobs that pay them less ✓.
  • Women have less media coverage and fewer role models to aspire to ✓ and less funding and sponsorship ✓.

  A range of social and economic barriers affecting women's participation in sport is given. Once again, more correct points are written down than there are marks available and Candidate B scores full marks.

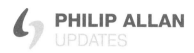
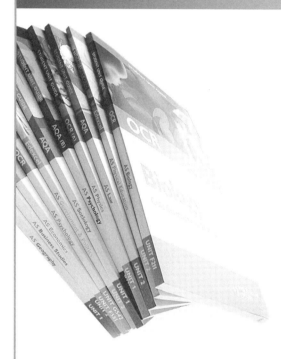